The Reality of Brain I

A respected medical professional, family man, and keen athlete, Andrew Tillyard had a full and active life until a vehicle crash changed it all. He sustained a serious head injury and was airlifted to the hospital where he worked, having only just survived. In this book, he recounts the raw, uncompromising struggles he faced to rebuild his life.

Drawing from regular blog entries written throughout his rehabilitation, Andrew provides an authentic reflection of the lived experience at some of the key stages along the road to recovery, from pragmatic concerns about new daily difficulties to wider concerns about his new place in life. He highlights the specific challenges and support he encountered as a person with a medical background who found themselves in a healthcare system as a patient. With frank honesty, he takes readers beyond the simple message that things can and do improve, by demonstrating that negativity, bitterness, and occasional rage are all necessary parts of the journey. However, he also describes the many little victories that helped him keep battling on, knowing there is always hope for the future. In particular, he narrates how he learnt to do things the doctors said he would never do: walking, reading, running, and ultimately writing this book. With the perspective of ten years since his injury, the book also charts a longer-term view of the ebb and flow of recovery.

This is essential reading for neuropsychologists, neurologists, and other rehabilitation therapists, as well as students in medicine, nursing, allied health, and neuropsychology. This is also a compelling and compassionate story for anyone who has survived a brain injury and who feels – as Andrew did at times – that life might not be worth living anymore, as it can show that there is always hope for the future.

Dr. Andrew Tillyard M.BChb, FRCA, EDICM was an Intensive Care Physician Consultant and Associate Professor of Medical Ethics and Law. Since his injury he has dedicated himself to finding a new life with meaning and ways to help others. This book is the next step in that process. Andrew is active on social media, and this book is largely based upon the blog (amistillmecom.wordpress.com) *Am I Still Me?*

After Brain Injury: Survivor Stories
Series Editor: Barbara A. Wilson

This new series of books is aimed at those who have suffered a brain injury, and their families and carers. Each book focuses on a different condition, such as face blindness, amnesia and neglect, or diagnosis, such as encephalitis and locked-in syndrome, resulting from brain injury. Readers will learn about life before the brain injury, the early days of diagnosis, the effects of the brain injury, the process of rehabilitation, and life now. Alongside this personal perspective, professional commentary is also provided by a specialist in neuropsychological rehabilitation, making the books relevant for professionals working in rehabilitation such as psychologists, speech and language therapists, occupational therapists, social workers and rehabilitation doctors. They will also appeal to clinical psychology trainees and undergraduate and graduate students in neuropsychology, rehabilitation science, and related courses who value the case study approach.

With this series, we also hope to help expand awareness of brain injury and its consequences. The World Health Organization has recently acknowledged the need to raise the profile of mental health issues (with the WHO Mental Health Action Plan 2013–20) and we believe there needs to be a similar focus on psychological, neurological and behavioural issues caused by brain disorder, and a deeper understanding of the importance of rehabilitation support. Giving a voice to these survivors of brain injury is a step in the right direction.

Titles include:
Life After My Mother's Stroke
A teenage take on how to cope
Tashi Hansen du Toit and Pieter du Toit

Reconstructing Identity After Brain Injury
A search for hope and optimism after maxillofacial and neurosurgery
Stijn Geerinck

For more information about this series, please visit: www.routledge.com/After-Brain-Injury-Survivor-Stories/book-series/ABI

The Reality of Brain Injury
Am I Still Me?

Dr. Andrew Tillyard

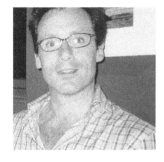

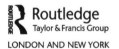

Routledge
Taylor & Francis Group

LONDON AND NEW YORK

Cover image: © Getty Images

First published 2022
by Routledge
4 Park Square, Milton Park, Abingdon, Oxon OX14 4RN

and by Routledge
605 Third Avenue, New York, NY 10158

Routledge is an imprint of the Taylor & Francis Group, an informa business

© 2022 Andrew Tillyard

The right of Andrew Tillyard to be identified as author of this work has been asserted in accordance with sections 77 and 78 of the Copyright, Designs and Patents Act 1988.

British Library Cataloguing-in-Publication Data
A catalogue record for this book is available from the British Library

Library of Congress Cataloging-in-Publication Data
A catalog record has been requested for this book

ISBN: 978-1-032-15503-6 (hbk)
ISBN: 978-1-032-15502-9 (pbk)
ISBN: 978-1-003-24437-0 (ebk)

DOI: 10.4324/9781003244370

Typeset in Times New Roman
by Apex CoVantage, LLC

For Bertie, Lila, and Florence – You each
are forever inspiring me forwards.

Contents

Acknowledgments

I think humour and kindness are vital for us all, and they have certainly played a big part in my journey towards recovery. So I would like to say thanks to everyone who has helped me on the way, showing their kindness and love, and for tolerating my humour, especially if you've ever been the butt of one of my jokes! And a very special thank you to all the lucky recipients of my occasional (constructive) sarcasm. I still maintain that it is a huge compliment to everyone who is on the receiving end; I'm making the assumption they have the ability to learn from my trenchant wit!

Thanks to Christopher Lomas for his help with this book.

Thanks to the Falmouth Cafe servers for putting up with me and laughing along with my jokes!

I apologize to you all for any un-woke language I may have used in this wrist-splitting diatribe! Thank you for reading.

Introduction

The temptation when asked to write this foreword was to describe my friend and colleague's heroic battle against adversity and his eventual 'winning' against the odds. In truth, Andrew would not recognise that character, neither would it acknowledge his current level of self-esteem. Regrettably for him, the battle is not over, the war not won, and when our subject frequently resorts to derogatory language to describe himself, the healing process is incomplete. What follows is an honest account by Andrew Tillyard of the life-changing brain injury he sustained whilst indulging his competitive instincts at a local triathlon. It describes his accident and the slow, tortuous route to his current level of function and ability. The words are his, based upon his recollections, his knowledge of trauma pathways, and his interpretation of conversations that have taken place. At times a tragic, poignant tale, it is also full of hope, Andrew's vernacular, and his unfettered wit. He has suffered many indignities since the crash, but he has retained the ability to laugh at himself, going some way to answering the question, 'Am I still me?'

At the time of his accident, Andrew was a happily married father of three small children, and that their family unit was unable to survive the sequelae of events remains a source of great sadness for all concerned. Despite the complexities of his disabilities and rehabilitation requirements, Andrew was

DOI: 10.4324/9781003244370-1

always supported by his wife and children, and they remain in close contact. Whilst he frequently reflects on his losses, this book is not a story of recriminations or what-ifs, but it describes one man's determination to reclaim his life and sense of self.

On the day in question, Andrew cycled headfirst into a camper van and was knocked unconscious by the collision. He was rapidly transferred to Derriford Hospital, Plymouth, where an acute subdural haematoma (ASDH) was diagnosed, and was then evacuated by the waiting consultant neurosurgeon. An ASDH is a potentially life-threatening bleed due to the pressure effects exerted upon the underlying brain tissues, but many patients go on to make a good recovery. Unfortunately, Andrew also had contusions (bruises) in both frontal lobes that continued to mature (swell). Furthermore, an artery supplying blood to the visual centres in his brain was blocked, resulting in a stroke. Swelling associated with the contusions and stroke provoked intracranial pressures that were dangerously high and threatened those areas of the brain that had not been damaged by the original blow. To relieve this, Andrew underwent a decompressive craniectomy, with surgeons removing part of the skull to allow the brain to swell without resistance from the cranial bones.

In total, he spent five weeks on the intensive care unit where, until recently, he had worked as a consultant. In medicine we understand that 'shit happens,' but nonetheless, it comes as an unpleasant surprise to treat one of your own, blurring those emotional boundaries that protect us when facing other people's misfortune.

A further 15 months passed in hospital and rehabilitation before Andrew returned home to Cornwall. During those first two years he was an in-patient in Plymouth and Bristol, where he required a shunt for hydrocephalus, a cranioplasty to replace the area of excised skull, and treatment for post-traumatic seizures. Against this background of medicalisation and rehabilitation, a normal life had to carry on, whilst family and friends adjusted to Andrew's disability, his cloak of capability, and the team of caregivers who entered their world. Visiting every few months I could see improvements in mobility, balance, and co-ordination, and when he lucidly asked about work colleagues and clinical problems, I assumed a greater degree of recovery than perhaps existed; this was his 'cloak.' Visitors could believe many things about the rate and extent of Andrew's restoration, but it was those closest to him who knew and understood the bigger picture, which existed beyond 'simple' functionality.

Prior to his accident, Andrew was a spectacle-wearing Australian but was otherwise fit and well. Physically, as an adult male he could do whatever he wished, and professionally he was ahead of the game. The crash changed that in an instant, with any subsequent progress being slow and hard-earned, requiring months and years to re-learn how to eat, drink, speak, read, write, walk, and run. As a friend I congratulate him on his progress, but he remains discontent because he could do all those things before, and nearing ten years post-injury he has been unable to return to work as an intensive care consultant and professor of medical ethics and law. The comedienne and broadcaster Ellen DeGenres (in her book, *Seriously . . . I'm Kidding*) has said, 'It is our flaws that make us human. If we can accept them as part of who we are, they really don't need to be an issue'. The painful reality for Andrew is that he acquired these flaws abruptly, without warning or preparation; he doesn't accept them; and he remains distressed by his loss of identity and ability.

Nonetheless, at the time of writing it is heartwarming to know that he has been in a relationship for 12 months and that his new partner embraces his character and foibles. Despite his despondency and frustration, this is a man who has a life worth living. He is loved by family and friends, has run a half marathon and completed a Tough Mudder, engages in public speaking, and writes poetry, a blog, and now this book. Andrew lives in his own apartment, and the 24-hour care has been reduced to drop-in sessions. Like many he finds great solace and peace of mind from a daily routine of exercise followed by coffee and cake. *The Reality of Brain Injury: Am I Still Me?* may be a difficult read for those facing similar problems, but I hope that you will be inspired by my friend's determination and desire to be the best version of 'me' that fate will allow.

Robin Berry, August 2021

1 How I Acquired My Brain Injury

The Triathlon

August 4th, 2012

Why did I have to do a triathlon on my wife's birthday? Somehow, I knew it was not going to play out well. But it was the local triathlon, and it would have seemed a shame not to take part. I'd been involved in helping to organise it, and I'd be back by one o'clock. . . . Well, that was the plan. I knew the kids would be desperate to celebrate by then, so we'd have a birthday lunch, and I'd give Liv her presents. What could possibly go wrong?

Outside, the sun was rising behind the church tower, and a warm August breeze came in through the bedroom window. As I lay in bed all I could hear was the sound of the cutlery barrage in the kitchen, signalling the coming of another food storm – breakfast for the kids, Bertie, Lila, and Florence! I shut out the thumps and roars of laughter and played over the possibilities for the race in my head. I was expecting a good finish; I wanted my son to see me do well after all the training that I had been putting in. I even thought it would be a good learning experience for him to see that hard work really did pay off.

I got myself ready, gulped down a quick breakfast, and kissed my wife and children goodbye. I loved them all, and I loved the life I lived with them. I was happy in my career, and to all intents and purposes, I felt invincible. Not for one second did I stop to consider the possibility that I might

DOI: 10.4324/9781003244370-2

leave that day and never go back to my family again. And yet everything that I knew and loved was going to be removed from me, not in one moment of madness but in a series of hundreds and hundreds of cuts.

I jogged out to my car, which was almost completely covered in pink cherry blossoms. On either side of the driveway, the last of the daffodils were still clinging to life and swayed in the gentlest of breezes. They seemed especially bright in their last flush of life. Inside the car, it was less picturesque. My wife used to refuse to get in there without some sort of CSI overalls to protect her from the discarded apple cores and orange peels, the mud- and cow-dung-encrusted welly boots, and the unmistakable presence of a sweaty, discarded running top stuffed in amongst all the other flora and fauna. I had to concede that it did resemble a bacterial growth-medium plate from the microbiology lab, but I wasn't interested in having a pristine status car; I just loved being busy, helping people, and enjoying my family and my life. I felt a shadow of guilt at leaving them that morning, but I'd be back by one.

Back by one. . .

On a normal day I would have already been well on my way to Treliske Hospital in Truro, where I was a Consultant Physician in Intensive Care. The job confronted me with new challenges every day, and I absolutely loved the work and knowing that I was helping so many people. I had endless energy in those days and always had dozens of projects on the go: I was researching pandemic flu, as well as being an Associate Professor of Ethics and Law, which meant I spent one day a week teaching and researching. And then when I got home after work, I was constantly planting new trees and building playhouses and zip slides in the garden for the kids. My wife had practically banned me from going to the garden centre because she said my projects were out of control.

The roads were quiet, and my mind eased back into race mode. I had been training incredibly hard, cycling every night after work and running in all weathers. I'd even bought a rowing machine to reduce the amount of training I had to do away from home. But I was still nervous about the swimming leg. I had never been the most confident swimmer, and to try to compensate, I had thrown money at the problem and bought myself a new wetsuit, or what I called 'my gimp suit'. After the swim, I knew I could make up ground in the cycle leg and hopefully take a bit of a lead into the running stage, giving me a good chance of finishing somewhere near the top.

Soon enough, I was standing on the start line with the rest of the gimps, looking like a scene from a weird arthouse film. I peered into the water nervously, keen to get going. Finally, the whistle blew, and off we went. I took in a big breath, ran down the beach to the water's edge, and carried on running as far as I could into the water before diving in. I was relieved to find myself in a position where I was relatively free of all the other competitors, so I didn't need to worry about getting kicked in the face – or somewhere worse!

The sandy seabed slowly receded as we hit deeper water, and I settled into a composed rhythm, just letting my body do what it needed to do to propel me through the water. I felt strong and knew I was out in the first group of triathletes, doing well.

At last, I could see the beach moving slowly – ever so slowly – closer, and I was still in among the leaders. I heaved myself out of the water, adrenaline pumping, and set off on the cycle leg in good spirits. I pushed my bike up the slipway and jumped onto it, powering up the long uphill section towards Rosevine. I felt fantastic on that bike; it was so light and fast, and I felt like I could outpace anyone.

In Tresillian, the route turned onto the main road from Tregony towards St Mawes and wound along a typical

Cornish country lane with high hedges, no verges, and a few too many blind corners. At the entrance to St Mawes, we hit a section of road with a long, gradual decline where you could work up quite a speed. Being a competitive bugger, I'm pretty sure I would have been giving it my all, going as fast as I possibly could. . .

But I can't remember any of that.

All I know of what happened next is pieced together from other people's recollections. Near the bottom of the hill, I hit a puddle and spun out of control, and when the camper van appeared unexpectedly around the blind corner, I crashed headfirst into it.

And that's when the drama really began. The rescue helicopter was on the scene in minutes, and I was loaded into a hard collar and flown up to the hospital in Derriford – the hospital I had been working in until quite recently. It would only have been five minutes or so later when I was handed over to a team of doctors and nurses. The paramedics would have given the lightening-speed handover they were used to: 'He's a mid-thirties male competing in a triathlon. He's suffered a serious head injury following an RTA. He's been unconscious but stable throughout the flight.'

I was intubated to help me keep breathing, and they got a size-14-gauge intravenous drip in, while keeping me as flat as a pancake. They didn't want me suddenly coughing or making an involuntary movement.

The Derriford team raced me, covered in emergency equipment now, into A&E, where I was quickly reassessed: Ventilation okay? Blood pressure stable? There would have been a tumultuous flurry of activity as the doctors and nurses all did their respective jobs, checking I was stable enough to be transferred to the emergency theatre, where a team of surgeons and nurses were already scrubbed and poised to begin operating.

Certainly, the anaesthetist and everyone else would have been relatively relaxed. I was quite a straightforward case; all they needed to do was to lift a large piece of damaged skull and remove the haematoma and any bit of the brain that had been damaged in the collision. It wasn't quite that straightforward, of course; they still had to ensure that there was not going to be too much fluid on the brain and that any fluid there was had a way to drain out, to prevent hydrocephalus – a dangerous swelling of the brain.

Of course, I was dead to the world, utterly unaware of any of it, but I can see it all happening in my mind's eye. I know so very well what would have happened and when, and I would have seen the same danger signs the anaesthetist saw. . . .

Hey presto, almost as if I wanted to ensure everyone was still awake, that's when I had a cardiac arrest. I know that would have put the willies up a few people, particularly the anaesthetist, who would have been cursing me as he tried desperately to get my heart going again. At the same time, the surgeon would have carried on operating on the small section of my exposed brain, oblivious to the anaesthetist running around like a blue-arsed fly. If anything, she was probably quite pleased with the bloodless field the cardiac arrest had caused – it made her work that little bit easier.

I'd been working on emergencies – just like my own – for five years at that very hospital, waiting, scrubbed up in the emergency theatre, for casualties to arrive. I'd be at the top end ready to anaesthetise poor buggers like me. I saw a few head injuries, and I knew the process well. The operation took about 45 minutes, after which I was wheeled off to intensive care – my very own ward – where I was greeted by a full-length picture of myself telling people: *If you cross the white line, wash your hands!* Not that I would have been at all recognisable, given my newly acquired, blood-stained turban and the coordinating jumble of medical equipment splayed all over me!

Once again, there would have been a recitation of my recent medical history, with a few new extras: 'It's predominantly a head injury, as best we can tell at this stage. He's had a C-scan, but his neck wasn't cleared definitively. Oh, and he had a cardiac arrest in theatre; his heart went into ventricular fibrillation, and he was given two shocks with the defibrillator.'

And so the nurses, Marc and Pierre (a German with a French name that I would go on to rib mercilessly when I got the chance, which wasn't immediately), set to work and got me settled into the ward. Whenever a new patient arrives in the ITU, the staff greet them with a certain exhausted, hangdog appearance; their overburdened workload has just got even heavier. And yet I know they would have set to work with diligence and professionalism, as always. Later, I heard they were all pretty upset to see me turn up in such a state. It's never great when a colleague suddenly becomes a patient.

By that time, my wife had arrived at the hospital and was greeted by the horrible sight of her husband in his blood-stained headwear and a sea of lines, drips, and emergency equipment. My parents were already heading for the airport in Melbourne to fly over to see me. Friends and family all over the place were mobilising, offering to help, to look after the children, to do something, *anything*.

All the while, I slept on, unresponsive. I slept on for nearly three weeks, blissfully unaware that I'd survived a life-threatening trauma to the head. And there was more to come. . . . The pressure on my brain kept increasing. Perhaps there was a torn vein or artery, but they needed to get back in there and remove a large piece of bone to relieve the pressure. That wasn't an ideal solution – recoveries tend to progress more smoothly without subjecting the head to even more disruption – but it was the best available solution.

(In case you're wondering, they later installed a titanium plate to replace the piece of skull they'd taken out. They usually 'bank' the removed piece of bone in the layer of fat in the abdomen; this keeps the bone in a viable state in case it's needed in the future for a bone graft. The problem was, I was just too fit. They couldn't find an ounce of fat on my abdomen, so they were unable to store it.)

So, cranial pressure building, you can imagine the panic among the anaesthetists over which one of them was going to give me the anaesthetic. They all knew me, of course, just as they knew that a few days earlier, when one of my old colleagues from the department had anaesthetised me, they'd had to shock me back into life when I went into cardiac arrest. I believe they ended up drawing lots to see who the unlucky anaesthetist was going to be.

I knew the surgeon very well, and she later told my parents, 'I half expected him to sit up after we'd finished and say, "Thanks Ann!"' But I stayed unresponsive. I couldn't say 'thank you' to any of them. The swift actions of the paramedics, the theatre staff, and the intensive care staff had saved my life. I'll be forever grateful to them all, to their quick reactions and professionalism. But little did I know that there were so many days to come, during the desperately slow and painful process of rehabilitation, when I would want to take my own life. Learning to talk and walk were only the beginning. Hardest of all was the realisation of the very different life that would face me when I woke up.

When I did wake after three weeks, I was kept under close observation for a further three weeks until I was finally moved from ITU onto a regular ward, six weeks after the accident. By God, my brain was so addled that I kept thinking I was in other parts of the country. Some mornings I found myself waking up in a hospital's secretary's office, or I was in an old flat in London or even in a future house in Cornwall. Sometimes I distinctly felt as if I had been walking along the beach with Olivia or we'd just been strolling down Bond Street on a Sunday afternoon. But then when reality kicked in, I was left with a sense of extreme sadness, not just because none of those things were true but because when she saw me, Liv didn't see her husband, she saw a patient in a hospital bed. Not even a man, but a vegetable; that's what they told her I was, and they said I would never be the same again.

Of course, I had never anticipated having such an unpleasant taste of my own medicine and arriving at the hospital I had been working in. Waking up to being a patient in what had been my very own ward, that was one hell of a hangover! Think about it – I had woken up in my own bed and travelled to the triathlon, and then the next thing I remember was being a cripple on my own ward. And at this point I should probably apologise for all my un-woke language, but you must see it from my perspective. . . . I had been a reasonably athletic Australian who woke up one morning to find himself completely disabled.

Most of those first few days and weeks are lost to me. But I remember the abject shock of being so suddenly rendered disabled and feeling as if I would never compete in a triathlon ever again. And yet that was the least of my worries; I felt I would never be able to walk or experience any kind of independence again. Worse, it seemed in those early days that I would be perpetually locked in my own mind, stuck forever in my wrecked body, unable to physically do anything, thinking constantly about what my life had been before the accident. Not without good reason, the experts in rehab and neurology were already thinking I should be pushed off to 'slow stream' rehab, or a nursing home.

One of my first reflections on my new situation might seem trivial to some, but I can assure you that you wouldn't think like that if you'd been in my shoes, or rather wheels.

Very quickly I realised: no one flirts with anyone in a wheel-chair. Later, I also discovered that one's ability to work at any sideboard was severely curtailed – it was impossible to get close enough because of the footrests – so I obviously wasn't going to be mixing any cocktails anytime soon.

I wasn't going to be engaging in much witty repartee either. They'd intubated me in ITU, and I was still struggling to speak. They tried me with a speaking valve in the 'trachy' tube and it didn't work. In a very muffled voice, I piped up as best I could, 'try another speaking valve!' They did, and it worked!

One of the most acute problems that I had to face first was not being able to use my left arm. I had always been pre-dominantly left-handed. I wrote with my left hand, held my tennis racquet with my left hand, and held my knife and fork the other way round to most people. (And I still got more food in my mouth than my children seemed to manage getting in theirs!) When I started school, I struggled so much to cut shapes with the scissors that my parents took me to a left-handed shop in Sydney to buy me some left-handed scissors.

I remember Liv bringing my son to see me in hospital. By then I was desperately trying to get my hand to work again. Liv would sit opposite me and tempt me with some dark chocolate, which she carefully placed on the other side of a very small table. They had travelled almost two hours in the car to see me, and I cannot tell you how desperate I was to show them some movement, any movement; even a bloody flicker would have been enough. More than any-thing, I wanted my son to see how helpful their coming to see me was. And I suppose I wanted to show Liv that I had embarked on the first steps of a full recovery.

But my left hand didn't respond. There was no flicker of movement. Just the agony of trying and failing to do some-thing so bloody simple. My failure to produce any movement for them left me in such an enormous state of self-loathing and resentment. I hated failing in front of my son, and so I retreated into myself, not properly able to express myself to anyone. I thanked them for coming and had to stop myself short of saying that I did not want them to come and see me anymore. Just thinking about it now brings me close to tears.

2 How I Coped Dealing with Carers

Living Life with the Scarers

Ironically, it was on an intensive care ward round as a trainee physiotherapist that I first realised I wanted to be a doctor. I can pinpoint the exact moment: I asked the person in charge of the trainees what the liver function tests were that all the doctors were talking about, and he, rather condescendingly, said, 'Don't worry about it, that is for the doctors to know.' I thought, *well, sod you!* I genuinely wanted to know, and it struck me that, rather than rooting around in the library for the answer, the easiest way to find out would be to train as a doctor. So that man's thoughtless condescension changed the course of my life irrevocably.

I might have thought twice about the whole enterprise if I'd known that to study medicine, I was going to have to travel halfway around the world to Glasgow. But, decision made, I left a sunny summer in leafy Melbourne for cold, wintry Glasgow. However, I do have to say that it was very friendly, and even quite civilised by Australian standards!

I chose Glasgow because a family friend lived there, but I was completely unprepared for what it would be like. *Glasgow, city of architecture*! they proudly proclaimed, but you could hardly make out the buildings behind the rainclouds. Or from underneath the umbrellas. But I worked hard to settle in. I signed up for some clubs – even if they all seemed to be indoor ones – film club, board games, etc. I also signed up

DOI: 10.4324/9781003244370-3

for the only outdoor club I found . . . windsurfing. Jesus. We had to chip the ice off our boards before we could even start.

Every raindrop made me homesick for Australia. But I started to make friends in Halls; there was Geordie John, a rock climber, who was chilled, long, and lanky. In the evenings we'd come back to the flat to find him hanging from the architraves. Giles was a vet; we used to play a lot of tennis together at the courts across the road. Perhaps we could have become members, it probably wouldn't have cost much, but we found that it was more fun to scramble over the fence. A bit of adrenaline to spice up the game. And there was Liv, this funny little hobbitty creature with her incredibly thick, ridiculous jerseys knitted by some South American tribe, all floral or covered in llamas in violent colours. There was really no excuse for them, not even the bitter cold.

Even I got inured to it eventually, as I made my way from university halls to the wards as a junior doctor. I remember vividly running around the wards with white coat, pagers, and multiple pens hanging off me. All done up in a long-sleeved shirt and tie, with my leather-soled shoes, sweltering in the heat of the hospital corridors. I remember a consultant sitting us down to congratulate us on taking the first step towards a long and productive career. Then he scanned the room and added that having lots of pagers was not a sign of importance, in fact it was quite the opposite! He did tell us we would soon get used to wearing an ever-so-slightly hangdog appearance from working late the night before. And of course, most of all, he reminded us of the absolute importance of listening attentively to the consultants when they dispensed their words of wisdom. Over and above everything else, I still remember the outright, unbridled fear at doing my first night on call and realising that I was essentially the backstop for every patient in the hospital.

I remember being a registrar in anaesthetics, the feeling of turning up to the next patient who was in a bit of a state, and seeing all of the other junior doctors turning to look at me with relief that I was there, and I would take charge, and that meant that everything would be okay. But then there were the surgical registrars and senior house officers, who could be the complete opposite. Some of them turned up with a significant degree of self-importance, matched only by their lack of understanding of their very own patients. My goodness, some of them were about as useful as a seamstress at a Velcro convention.

We gave the surgeons a bit of a tough time, but of course we realised that it would be quite useful to be able to put everything back together again after you had chopped out whatever bit of offending body part it was that you were removing. And so, accordingly, a significant part of our training was directed to stitching everything back together again. I couldn't be bothered with all of that, though. I was far more interested in diagnosing the origin of a patient's illness rather than stitching everything back together again; I mean, I was not a seamstress! Ever so slowly, I rose up the training ladder of intensive care and anaesthetics. It felt like a very comprehensive training regimen, where one felt like one could do everything that the consultants were doing. My own rise to the level of consultant necessitated an interview with ten or more people, all sitting around a table, and I remember never quite knowing how I was supposed to look at everyone when I was giving my answers.

Unsurprisingly, one of my most abiding memories of those days was of a patient whose life we had collectively saved on the intensive care unit. All he could say was how unhappy he was that the surgeons had not sewn up his skin precisely enough, so that the huge, outstretched wings of an eagle tattooed on his chest were uneven. The irony that he was in any position to be able to complain about that – or indeed, to complain about *anything* – was sadly lost on him.

For balance, I do also remember cocking up completely when I was working on a cardiology ward and rushing around like all the other junior doctors did. We had patients coming in with infective endocarditis, which meant we had to prescribe a small truckload of antibiotics for each patient. I remember gathering up every patient's drug chart on the ward – that was the most efficient way to do all of the drug prescriptions – and I remember confusing one patient's chart for another. I prescribed penicillin, despite there being a warning, written in very large red letters: allergic to penicillin! Thank God the nurses began their drugs round late that day and we were able to sort it all out.

*

I had a lot of time to think back over my past when I was in recovery. And I often thought about those cold days in Glasgow. . . . Perhaps it had something to do with the ground-breaking ultra-cooling technique that they used on me in hospital. In hindsight, I know that I was lucky to be enrolled in the treatment arm of the therapeutic hypothermia study. In their work with other patients with traumatic brain injuries they had started collecting evidence that cooling the body down to just 32 degrees Celsius could help the brain recover more completely in the very early phases. My parents told me that I looked like a pharoah with the ice cooling bags covering my body and draped around my head like an Egyptian headdress. The theory goes that the brain gets less active at lower temperatures; in lay terms, it goes into a kind of hibernation and so requires less oxygen and fewer nutrients. Now I do know that one's brain isn't exactly doing a crossword when one is in a medically induced coma, but just think about sleep. . . . When you sleep, your brain stays very active to take care of a whole lot of basic housekeeping tasks it's required to do, such as keeping you breathing and keeping your heart beating. But if we can switch off these brain activities, then all the nutrients and activity that would otherwise be going on in the brain can be directed to helping it recover from the injury.

I don't know to what extent that process helped my eventual recovery, but I do think it's entirely fair to say that – in more ways than one – the NHS has been responsible for me still being here today. I can go further: the NHS – more than any one person – has been more responsible for making me who I am today. I'm not trying pass the buck here, or pass the blame (even I need to accept a modicum of responsibility for me!). It's all too easy to denigrate the NHS, but in reality, if it were not for the staff who love what they do – and very often go above and beyond what their contracts say they 'should' be doing – then the whole NHS would grind to a halt.

I certainly put my NHS colleagues to the test over those first few weeks after I was admitted. You may remember that I mentioned the danger of hydrocephalus earlier, and sure enough, I was well on my way to getting a soggy brain and needed an op to have a shunt inserted. One of the signs of hydrocephalus is an unsteady gait, something that anybody who knew me in the early stages of my recovery would have noticed as I bobbed and weaved unsteadily about the place. Another delightful sign of hydrocephalus is urinary incontinence, and I had that too. On the day my well-to-do father-in-law came to see me in hospital, they got me dressed in adult-sized nappies! Suffice to say, I was mortified. While I managed not to die of embarrassment, it seemed that some people thought I was ready to be shuffled off somewhere else to die of irrelevance. There were further complications from the hydrocephalus, and, indeed, my recovery might have taken an altogether smoother path without it, so by the spring of 2013, it was being suggested that I should go to a 'slow stream' rehab facility, potentially en route to a nursing home.

I'm told that both Liv and my mother petitioned the specialist in charge to have me admitted to Frenchay, in

Bristol, a 'fast track' rehabilitation hospital. They still believed I had it in me to achieve more. At that stage, I just needed to be able to be transferred from the bed into a wheelchair with only one person helping me. If we could get to that stage, then I would be allowed to go home, rather than the slow route to obsolescence in the nursing home.

Of course, the specialist could hardly refuse two such spirited requests from two such committed and eloquent women, and they finally agreed to take me to Frenchay for three months.

I was transferred to Bristol on 15th May 2013, and my parents had come over from Australia and rented a flat nearby, just so they could be close to their errant son and heir. My memories of those first few months range from hazy to impenetrable. In addition to the trauma of the collision, the encephalitis buggered my memory up even more! But I'm told that I ended up staying five months instead of three.

I essentially had to re-learn how to use every single muscle in my body. I couldn't even hold my head up at first. I think some newborn babies would have been giving me a race to see which of us could figure it out first! But bear in mind that my own head would weigh about ten pounds!

One of the highlights of staying at Frenchay was undoubtedly the time when we all had to evacuate. It was the height of summer, temperatures had soared to a seemingly unprecedented British high of 32 degrees, and we all had to wheel, limp, or crawl to our fire assembly point outside so we could wait in the baking sun. Then I had to go and do my special extra work that my parents had arranged with a specialist Neurophysiotherapist and Bobarth Tutor and we relocated to a little tin portacabin where we boiled until we emerged like pink lobsters. It was almost as if I was being punished with extreme heat for being Australian.

While I was at Frenchay, I was proudly presented with the answer to all my prayers: unlimited and unrestricted freedom of movement in . . . an electric wheelchair! The electric wheelchair was the last great hope of everyone around me, and what a joke that turned out to be. If nothing else, it did at least make me realise that I would have to become fully independent ASAP if I ever wanted to get anywhere ever again. Once home, and on a good day with a fair wind, I tried to put the thing through its paces. I would manoeuvre myself to the top of the sloping driveway and set off at top speed, with my parents running after me, begging me to slow down. It looked like a group of geriatrics chasing after Stephen Hawking while he was high on speed. Not the sort of thing you'd see too often in the Cornish countryside. Now, when I say 'top speed' I mean as fast as I possibly could, but that damn chair was no Formula One vehicle. Indeed, I think there was one occasion when my more-or-less 80-year-old father was walking beside me quite happily, if not overtaking me. Of course, by the time we got to the bottom of the hill, the bloody battery had run out of charge in its efforts to carry me down the slope, and my poor parents had to hurry back up the hill to fetch me a manual wheelchair. As you may have found out for yourself, electric wheelchairs are almost impossible to push manually, and it seemed like you need a small industrial forklift to replace the battery!

The electric wheelchair experiment didn't last long, and I was given a bog-standard manual number. I'm sure that manual wheelchairs are a useful tool for people who have one or even two good hands and arms at their disposal. I had a right hand that was about as effective as most people's left hand and a once-dominant left hand that was about as effective as a cotton glove in pool of piranhas.

Inevitably, I do remember the grand occasion of my release from Frenchay. I felt like a prisoner being let back out into the community. I didn't have an electronic tab so they could keep track of my whereabouts, but having seen me in my manual wheelchair, it wasn't as if I would have poised much of a flight risk. My memories of being delivered home in the wheelchair van and being delivered to my front door are even more distinct. It was October 13th, nearly 15 months after my accident. There were still some late summer flowers out to greet me, but it was all a far cry from the triumphant return I'd envisaged after my triathlon. I wasn't returning as the all-conquering hero; I was returning as a man who was learning to steer a wheelchair.

I seemed to spend hours upon hours in the kitchen, which was quite large, and I couldn't even get from one end to the other in my wheelchair because I kept veering off to the left. It didn't matter how hard I practised, and by God, I did practise, although some might say I was mostly practising my swearing or consolidating some deeply negative thoughts in my inner monologue. But the frustration was intense, and it felt at times as if it would break me.

I tried over and over again to get my damn chair just to move from one end of the kitchen to the other. The chair was, after all, supposed to give me back some small sense of independence, but all it did was exaggerate my sense of ineptitude. There I was, supposedly in the prime of my life, and I couldn't even get a stupid wheelchair to move. I was so deeply depressed that I had gone from competing in a triathlon to sitting in a chair that I seemed to be incapable of moving on my own.

It's fair to say that my mental health had been better! I spent so much of my time over days and weeks just sitting in that damn chair, alone and silent, trapped in my own mind, and that wasn't a very pleasant place to be. When I mustered enough enthusiasm to have another go, I veered off and hit the wall again. And then I would have another go and hit the wall again. And again. So, it went on, day after miserable day, as my energy and motivation just drained away.

It wasn't the physical exhaustion – I could hardly move, after all – but it was the mental strain of everything that had happened and the dawning realisation of the hell my life had become. The steady drip, drip, drip of one disappointment after another leached away at me. I hated knowing that I was just making the same mistakes in the wheelchair – and in everything else I tried to do – over and over again. It wasn't as if I was actively doing it wrong on purpose, but the sense that my body was never going to be able to do what was being asked of it was crushing. There was nothing I could simply change about what I was doing, and I felt as if it didn't matter how often I tried or how hard I worked at it; nothing was going to change. Nothing was going to improve.

By God, I bet I was insufferable in those first few days and weeks after getting home. It wasn't just the sheer desperation of my situation, there was something potentially worse in store for me. . . . Suddenly I had to share most of my life and seemingly my every waking moment with carers . . . or 'scarers' as I preferred to call them! Oh, and that took some adjustment.

In all seriousness, it is absolutely vital that you develop some form of relationship with your carers. It took a little while for me to make the adjustment to living with strangers, but, despite my ribbing, they were all good people, and I even managed to forge a decent working relationship with each and every one of them, even our Mr Biscuit. He called himself a chef. I should have known never to trust a skinny chef, but when the scarer whom I shall forevermore call Mr Biscuit offered to cook our turkey, he cooked it until it was as dry as a biscuit. I should point out that whilst cooking the bird, he frequently acknowledged how turkey meat could often be very dry when cooked and even went so far as to tell me about the many and varied ways one can ensure that one's turkey does not dry out too much, none of which he used while the oven blasted our poor bird to complete dryness. I'm no chef, but I prefer the more reliable method: you keep checking it as you go along and perhaps even slightly undercook it. Provided you're sure you have a full supply of loo roll in the house, you'll have a not-dry bird.

Then there were the gullible scarers, one of whom was so credulous that I had him believing that my very gentle and reserved parents were going off to get tattoos before enjoying an evening out watching the cage fighting. And I managed to persuade the other that one of my carers, who was originally from South Africa, had chosen to have one leg amputated because the government was giving away free Oscar Pistorius blades to anyone who was willing to volunteer for amputation (in an effort to boost the medal tally for the South African team at the Paralympics, obviously). I hope you'll indulge me in allowing me to tell you about my little games. As I'm sure you know very well, you have to find whatever ways you can to keep your sanity.

Meanwhile I carried on in my efforts to master the finer points of getting from A to B without having to go via D, E, and F in the wheelchair. Getting to grips with basic forward momentum and the occasional three-point turn was one thing, but it was quite another whenever I tried to survive outside the protective cocoon of its cold embrace, and I couldn't even be relied upon to stand up without falling over.

Of course, I spent a fair bit of time with occupational therapists (OTs), who are essentially there to help you work around whatever physical difficulties you have suddenly been faced with as a result of your accident or injury. For example, if you're having trouble walking, they would arrange for you to have a wheelchair. Because I had trouble with a lot more than just walking, they provided me with a range of specialist equipment, including a set of chopping boards to help me cut up all those vegetables and some specially adapted cutlery to help me eat. There was even a surprisingly comfortable, motorised lounge chair that I could lie back in and put my feet up. In fact, of all the equipment that I received that's the one I still use most today.

One of my OTs was very pleased with herself when she presented me with an enormous, inflatable double-bed-sized thing. I was supposed to roll back onto it whenever I fell over and could not get back up again. And it was always *when* I fell, not *if.* It would be the ultimate understatement to suggest that I fell *quite* often; I fell over all the bloody time in those days. There were Olympic divers in training who dived less than I did. It was a miracle that I was ever on my feet for more than a few seconds. And let me tell you, I weighed a tenth of a ton in those days, so it would have taken a team of weightlifters to hoist me back to my feet before I inevitably wobbled and hit the floor again. The mattress was supposed to make it easier to get some leverage so I could bring myself back up again. But it was so big and cumbersome even when it was entirely deflated, and the scarers were supposed to carry around the enormous double-bed-sized-mattress suitcase that it came in. They would have needed the strength of Arnold Schwarzenegger to take it wherever I had fallen so that I could get up without hurting them.

Then there was the enormous inflatable condom thing that I was supposed to wear on my left arm. The air in the condom was supposed to be a gentle way to help me straighten it out. Otherwise, it was permanently bent up against my shoulder. It seemed as if the only thing that was not an inflatable was the root cause of all of my issues, my damn brain. Perhaps there was enough air billowing around in there already.

3 How I Started to Find Inspiration After My Brain Injury

The Pathetic Limping Tillyard Charity

Over the four years we worked together, my physiotherapist said she had never had a patient quite as motivated to get better as me. But God, it was bloody hard work. Physiotherapy is, of course, all about getting your body to work again, which means making it work against the new limitations the brain injury has put upon you. You essentially have to convince your body to learn how to move in new ways in order to complete a task. It's bloody difficult work when you're having to try and learn a movement that before your brain injury would have made sense, but after brain injury seems like some weird, alien choreography with limbs that don't want to cooperate. What is colloquially known as muscle memory is thrown out of the window. I already knew a fair bit about what was going to be in store for me when I met the physios, as I had obtained a degree in physiotherapy in Australia before I went to Glasgow.

After 15 months of rehab in hospital and ongoing work with the physiotherapist at home, I got to a point where I could sort of walk, but not in a way that would convince anyone that I wasn't liable to fall over at any second. I had my suspicions that my carers were under strict instructions that I should not be allowed to walk anywhere unobserved. Of course, that just led to me coming up with a whole heap of spurious fools' errands requiring them to go over to the barn so that I could get up and walk to the other end of the

DOI: 10.4324/9781003244370-4

kitchen, which looked larger and larger with every teetering step I took. Or I would walk in the playroom in front of the three-seater sofa, so that if I fell down, I would have a soft landing.

Now, when I say 'walking' it was really just coordinated limping! But I still sent the carers away so that I could build up my confidence in walking unaided, rather than with the handling belt which was designed so a scarer could support me if needed while I was tottering along. When I was off the reins, so to speak, I gravitated to wearing an American-style gridiron sports helmet to protect the hole in my head. I'm not sure how useful it was, given that it was intended to protect something (a brain) that I no longer had anyway! Without the helmet, my mother said you could sometimes see the pulsing movement of my brain beneath the hollow where that piece of skull had been.

I used to wear that helmet whenever I was out of my wheelchair, even if it was just for a little trip to the GP's surgery. And then I would sit in the waiting room, looking like a disabled child with my special helmet on.

Ideally, they'd have covered over the hole as soon as possible, but, as they told Liv, there was a chance I might not survive the op. She decided it would be better to let me come home for a while first so that I could spend some time with my family. I had already survived the crash and the cardiac arrest, so she must have thought that it would be third time unlucky!

So it was nearly two years after the accident when I went in to have a titanium plate fitted. If Liv was nervous, I was even more acutely aware of what could go wrong. I remembered doing the anaesthetics for a chap who was having the same operation, and sadly, he did die. (I hasten to add that he did not die because of anything I did or didn't do!) But it obviously weighed heavily on my minuscule brain, and having signed a new will and said my reluctant goodbyes to my wife and my kids, I went on one last walk around my beautiful house and gardens before leaving for the operation. The last time I'd said formal goodbyes to them all had been before the triathlon; I hoped earnestly that they weren't hours away from receiving more bad news about my fate on the operating table. Even then, I reflected on the strangeness of my situation and how, having so little of my brain left, I was still able to manage to feel the full range of human emotions.

One of the hardest things for me to deal with, apart from feeling so enfeebled, was feeling so beholden to my scarers. I know they all worked incredibly hard just to try and help me get my life back on track, so I felt as if I owed it to them – as well as myself – to strive for every little incremental improvement. With my buggered body striving to work against its new limitations, two hours of exercise a day seemed woefully insufficient on its own. I got my scarers to help me do more, and I found that it was helpful to marshal them into different groups, so they could help with different exercises and activities that best reflected their different abilities. When they all knew the exercises I needed to practise and could help in ways that made it easier for me, it helped me to work with sustained commitment.

I found the very best inspiration to go on improving came in the unlikeliest places; a friend from Glasgow came down to stay with me, and during his visit, I fell over the table. In the old days he would have said, 'Get up, you clumsy bugger!' But now he was being so kind to me, so sympathetic, and God, I was embarrassed, mortified even. The phrase I coined to describe his new touchy-feely attitude was 'positively negative'. It's the same phrase I used to describe my attitude to rehab exercises. But you take your inspiration where you can, and for me, there was no better motivation to go on exercising and go on pushing myself. Never mind all the great times we'd had together as friends in the past – those didn't help me a jot. All I had to do was think about the moment that I fell over. Whenever I thought of that, it forced me on with the physio: another step, and another, and another. . . . It was never quite that straightforward, of course. Sometimes the motivation outstripped my capacity to exercise, and I worked so hard and got so tired I couldn't focus any more.

I had been left with a huge bag of issues, sure enough, but the tiredness was among the worst of them. I sometimes felt as if I had been left with one, single, solitary functional neuron, and the poor thing was working overtime. As a result, I felt exhausted all of the time. Such simple things as meeting new people or just going somewhere different – i.e. anything out of the ordinary – was enough to leave me feeling utterly done in. It was the same sort of exhaustion I used to get after I had studied for a very long time. Depressingly, it seemed to be utterly intractable, but practise – and lots of it – was key.

The more I practised everything, the more the tiny victories stacked up, even if they did all seem utterly insignificant. They were hardly the sorts of things that were going to win me a medal or get my picture in the paper. And as far as anyone else would be concerned, they must have seemed like the littlest of little life tasks, the sorts of things that most people take for granted. But increasingly, I knew that they were exactly the sorts of things that really illustrated just what I had to overcome.

My balance was still completely shot, and it was so unbearably awful that if you came looking for me at any point in those early days, there was a more than even chance that you'd have found me lying on the floor, having fallen over in some ignominious place yet again. It took an Olympian feat of effort to get myself off the ground after a fall. And yes, I really was like one of those giant Galapagos tortoises who was lying on his back, and at the time, I felt as if I weighed about a tenth of a ton too!

I seemed to spend an inordinate amount of time on the ground. It almost always seemed to happen if I was trying to impress someone with my newfound proficiency too. *Look what I can do . . .* crash. *Bugger.* But every tiny building block enabled me to move on to even more complex tasks like – drumroll, please – loading and unloading the dishwasher! The very best way to practise anything – especially balance – was to focus on a standard daily task. At first, I still needed someone to stand beside me while I actually loaded or unloaded it. Miraculously, I only dropped one of my beautiful Ricard Bramble plates. In my new world of reduced proficiency, that felt like a win.

I do need to point out that progressing from immobile chair-bound doughnut through proficient dishwasher operative to a relatively normal-seeming, independent adult took time. A hell of a lot of time. Reading about it here in the space of 40,000 words or so can't possibly do justice to the time and effort it took, and it can never quite convey the amount of blood, sweat, and tears involved. Just be thankful you don't have to read about every slip and fall and setback, because there were so very many. If you've been through this journey yourself, you'll know only too well. Just as you'll know that even in the littlest of victories, there are the seeds of other bigger victories. What started out as a daily slog of balancing and articulating myself in the most ungainly ways just to get the ruddy things in and out of the dishwasher actually became almost satisfying in itself, as I slowly, slowly saw the incremental improvements. There really is nothing better than signs of improvement to keep spurring you on. I remember almost racing to eat my dinner just so that I could get back to the ongoing challenge of doing the dishwasher. And yes, that statement is simultaneously one of the most tragic and one of the most inspiring things I have ever said!

The point is that it can be hard to see the little victories in isolation, but just like my dishwasher, they do start to stack up. The day that I was able to go solo without my balancing aid scarer was, in its own way, a great day. A victory. Not quite on a par with victory at the Battle of Waterloo, perhaps, but a victory nonetheless.

I realised that progress was a one-step-forwards-two-steps-backwards kind of thing sometimes. Nothing proceeds in a straight line. Talking of which, walking got harder as I got better at it. By which I mean taking those first few faltering steps was one thing; stringing them together was much harder. Something as simple as walking a few paces in a straight line now required my absolute attention on every single step. It wasn't just a question of when to move my right foot or when to move my left but of thinking about each component of every movement. I had to ensure that I got my heel to strike the ground first, which also meant ensuring I extended (or dorsiflexed) my ankle and lifted my toes, but not too much or they wouldn't contribute anything to my balance or stability. Likewise, I also needed to gently plantarflex my ankle and let my foot touch the floor during mid-stance, so that my foot was flat and getting the most contact with the ground so as to aid my balance during the stance phase. I had to remember to bend my knee slightly – but not too much – when my heel struck the ground. Then there was the propulsion phase, and I had to ensure I was rolling over my left foot and getting into position with my right foot and toes so they were ready for the push-off with my calf, which should also be contracting in readiness. . . . Simple, eh?!

In addition to that, I also had to concentrate unnaturally intensively on the other senses I was getting from my ankle, foot, and knee. And all the while I was trying to do all of that *and* remember what to do next, I was expected to hold a conversation too!

My useless brain played all sorts of tricks on me, trying to convince me that what I was being told was correct was actually utterly abnormal. The best example of that was my brain telling me that I was standing upright, when, in fact, I was leaning a jaunty 30 degrees to the left. (You didn't need to be Einstein to work out why I was so fond of falling to the left.) Imagine a tall man loping along the street, all super-relaxed and lanky – like Shaggy in the *Scooby-Doo* cartoons – that's what my walking gait used to look like. Even after I managed to correct my leaning posture, I still felt as if the problem persisted. Whenever I was up and walking, it seemed to me as if I was wobbling and wavering all over the place, and I still felt as if I was being pulled strongly to my left and backwards, despite that not being the case and despite the constant reassurances that I was standing and walking dead straight.

I had to learn to try and ignore it, but the pulling sensation was incredibly strong, and my disordered muscles were firing in such a way that made me feel they were resisting my every move. It just didn't matter how many times people told me I was moving freely, I still felt the pull backwards whenever I tried to move forwards. To mitigate it, I limited my turning and reduced my stride length. Essentially, I altered my walking pattern to accommodate my perceived failings as a human walker, and by God, my failings were effing legion! The physio helped me learn how to use muscles again – and use them in the right way – so that I wasn't forever destined to look like a cartoon character.

Now under normal circumstances, there are neurons that fire to stimulate the muscles that need to work to complete the movement. But then you also have a series of other muscles that contract at the same time in order to help create a stable base from which you can complete the movement, and it was those muscles that were contracting so strongly, such that I felt I had suddenly inherited a heap of somebody else's muscles, each one resisting my every move. I used to call them my female muscles, and the reason I called them that is because I am Australian – I think you'll be getting used to my less than politically correct Aussie humour now – and my muscles just used to do whatever the bloody hell they wanted to do! Of course, I knew that my disordered muscles were responding to my frazzled brain. But my brain was about as useful as a chocolate oven glove, and it kept sending down signals to make the muscles contract even though I didn't want them to contract.

My sister, Jane, is a trained neurological physiotherapist and a Bobath specialist. Very simply, the Bobath approach was developed to help manage neuromotor dysfunction in children with cerebral palsy. It's designed to promote the sensory and motor pathways and encourage normal muscle control and movement, rather than relying on compensatory movements. Whenever she came to see me, it didn't take her long to point out all of the problems I was having with my locomotion. She put me on a training programme to help me make my movement more efficient. Once again, it was all about the balance, and I did find it amazing how important having good balance is for just about everything. Even though I had two good legs, I found out that it is how well we stand on just one leg that provides a key marker of how well we will walk and turn.

The work could be excruciatingly painful at times, because any sensation I did get in my leg felt wrong at first. However, I was accumulating a degree of sick pride in seeing how far I had come from my accident, and that did help me to see my progress more clearly. Jane had heard all of the same things the so-called experts said to my wife and family about how I would end up in a persistent vegetative state, hardly able to do anything more inspiring than raise a cocked eyebrow or two, and for a long time afterwards, I felt so cheated of the life that I thought had been denied me. But with her help and the ongoing support of the scarers, I made steps and then strides forwards.

My parents also enlisted the help of a specialist physio teacher of Bobath therapy, as practised by my sister. It was hard trying to relearn all of these once-familiar movements after my body had been dulled by lack of proper use. You're not just re-learning how to chop a carrot or hold a tennis racquet; you're learning how to do those things in the right way. You mustn't fall into the trap of overcompensating for the lack of use by adopting techniques which may feel easier in the short term but which will only make life harder in the long term. I continued with the Bobath therapy for seven years, having occasional sessions of concentrated treatment over the course of several days at a time. So if you see me leaning to one side now, maybe it's because you're listing to 30 degrees, not me.

But even when I started to show the buggers wrong, I had no way of knowing how much I could improve or how long I would be in the living hell of only ever being able to move so very clumsily. As much as any Australian could ever be described as elegant, I was the epitome of inelegance. There was no suppleness or spontaneity in my movement, so that when the kids came over for the afternoon and wanted to play in the park, I tried but couldn't join in. It wasn't as if it was a game of subtle movement and precision; they were playing tag, and all I could do was watch because I was so worried about falling over. Whenever I tried to make any quick, spontaneous movement, my knee stiffened up and I could only limp. And it was a slow, ungainly limp at that.

Even as my normal walking began to improve (over uncountable hundreds of hours of hard work) I continued to walk with a barely perceptible sway, and I really had to concentrate hard to carry off any illusion of normality. For the most part, I felt like a tightrope walker, wavering all over the place, straining every sinew to walk ever so carefully, step by tentative step. It really did feel as if I was balancing very precariously on each leg as I stepped from left to right, right to left. And there wasn't ever a safety net to catch my fall or even any applause for safely navigating the next step.

It might have passed muster in the big top, but in the children's playground where there were obstacles everywhere – particularly other people's children – I looked and felt out of place. Not that anyone who knew me would have thought so. They were all quick to praise the progress I'd made, but they weren't the ones who had to sit on the sidelines and watch while their children played without them being able to join in. All I wanted to do was to play with my children; it didn't feel like too much to ask.

For anyone reading this hoping to find out my top tip on surviving or coping with a brain injury, it would be . . . TO NOT HAVE ONE! However, I do think my deeply rooted and genuine love of a challenge helped me engage with it all and learn to love walking again. Even when I began to realise just how fucked up I was after the accident, I started to think it was good that I had so much work to do! With so many different things to work on, I knew I'd never get bored. . . . But it turned out that I was wrong about that, and I soon realised just how boring it was to continually be working on the same mundane – but difficult – things just in an effort to be me!

The rest of me wasn't looking too promising, either; I still had my speech to work on, and my writing, which was not helped at all by the bastard club of a hand that I had been left with. And yet I knew that I was objectively so much better than I had been the last time I had reviewed my progress, just as I knew, deep down, that I was *still* improving, even if it did require monumental effort and endless extra work just to make it appear if I was functioning normally. I felt as if I had to metaphorically yell at my body to get it to carry out the simplest of movements. Raising my foot off the ground or waggling my thumb required such determined decisions that they excluded any other thinking. And so I found that it was easier to do things in complete silence – even with a degree of sensory deprivation – which is hard with young children with seemingly Olympian energy levels and impatience to match.

Outside of rehab, 'real life' carried on as best it could. The children weren't about to change into quiet, timid little creatures just for my benefit. But the juxtaposition between my two worlds seemed to be growing as wide as the distance between husband and wife. Even as we drifted apart, there were moments – little moments, usually – that gave me something to hang on to. Perhaps in an effort to keep that semblance of real life hanging on, Liv used to drag me out shopping with her. Shopping was always one of my least favourite activities, but I did feel more like myself when we had some time on our own together. I remember the last trip we took into St Mawes together, in a howling gale, joking as we went that we should set up a charity – the Pathetic Limping Tillyard charity, perhaps?!

Food was one of the few pleasures that remained to me, which is why I had to be so careful about what – and how much – I ate. Liv told me I had to lose weight to make it easier to move around, and she was right, of course. But on the other hand I had to have some enjoyment in life. And I was at least lucky in that respect; some people do lose their senses of taste and smell after an injury like mine. (I often wondered why we need a sense of smell to be able to taste, particularly given that some of the most disgusting-smelling foods such as Camembert – it smells like the skin of a peeled rabbit – can also taste so fantastic.) Two of my scarers, Arran and Jerry, were trained chefs, unlike Mr Biscuit, and regularly filled the house with tempting aromas, so I was particularly thankful that I had not lost my sense of smell or taste.

But my word, the human body is so precisely organised and ordinarily, the multitude of functions it carries out in the background keep us ticking along so seamlessly. But it just takes the smallest perturbation to bring it all down like a pack of cards and knock it off course. I had lost so much sensation in my mouth, and because I was so paranoid at the prospect of looking like a drooling idiot, I stopped opening my mouth fully, and I didn't enunciate my words very clearly.

I took some medication to dry up my excess secretions of saliva, but that left me with an incredibly dry mouth. So much so that it made it nigh-on impossible to eat scones. Imagine living in Cornwall and not being able to eat scones! I found this out to my great disappointment when I travelled to my favourite café, and my dry mouth rendered me completely unable to swallow my scone. Indeed, I was in very serious danger of suffocating. Forget waterboarding, I experienced near-death by scone. Of course, I did what any red-blooded Australian would do and blamed the chef and the café. Clearly, they had not cooked my scone properly. Sadly, they had not been to the same waiting school that I'd attended as a kid doing weekend jobs, and instead of sympathising and offering free scones for life, they gave me pretty short shrift.

The scarers were more accommodating of my moods and even allowed me to chip in and help out with some of their cooking, and I particularly enjoyed being able to make profiteroles with them, Bertie's favourite pudding. But when lunch was over or the cooking things had been put away, I usually found myself stuck in the same tired routine of just sitting and waiting for the next thing to happen. I had been such a hyperactive person before. My whole personality had been predicated on doing things, but in those days, tired of every morning's exertions, I just sat for long, lonely hours each afternoon. I could see that I needed to formulate other ways of having fun, but I hadn't come up with many. I supposed that I was probably depressed. Anti-depressants had been suggested to me, but I didn't want to take them because they weren't ever going to be able to treat the cause, were they? They would only ever have been able to treat the symptoms. I felt that I needed to be independent for the depression to lift.

The evenings were the worst time of all. The kids invariably came back from school tired and irritated, and they were cheeky to Liv. I used to try and tell them off, but they didn't listen. They were just being normal kids, growing up fast, but I felt so angry because I just had to sit there and observe it; they never paid any attention if I tried to intervene.

When it was a one-on-one, I found that we connected better. I tried to play games with them, and sometimes Bertie and I would talk about science, while Lila liked to draw and make things. . . . Florence wasn't really aware of what was going on. It was normal for her to have me sitting there. But as everyone got more and more tired, it felt as if the evenings would descend into farce. I felt like the Steve Martin character, Ruprecht, in *Dirty Rotten Scoundrels*, and so every day would end with the scarers taking me back to my barn at about 9.15. I was already desperate to get to bed by then, desperate to get away from them.

Perhaps you understand that feeling? Perhaps you know just what it's like to be required to have such an intimate relationship with a team of people you never knew before? Despite my teasing, they were kind people, they were really good at their job – and I know how hard that job must have been – but we hadn't chosen to become friends. It felt like an arranged marriage. Even when it felt like we were getting on really well, it could be hard to escape a sense of powerlessness and even resentment. More than that, I used to feel so inadequate around them.

So, at the end of every exhausting, inadequate day, I fell asleep alone, hoping against hope that the following morning, I would somehow, miraculously, be better.

4 How My Marriage Fell Apart After My Accident, And How I Came to Terms with It

Bricks in the Wall

It was another cracker of a day in Falifornia – as I like to call Falmouth – a glorious winter's morning. The sun was slowly rising above the horizon, a bright orange slither separating the increasingly bright blue of the sky from the moody azure-blue of the sea in the distance. I was already out, running, thinking about the course my life had taken, thinking about the things that had held me back and the things that had spurred me on. . . .

I had progressed through my formal physical rehab like a dazed deer on roller skates, through tentative walking to jogging and eventually to running, but I was still having huge perceptual problems, such as manoeuvring between chairs in a restaurant. And I still had a lack of sensation in one hand which made any dexterous task next to impossible. Because I couldn't feel it working, I found that I had to look at my hand or see my fingers to know what they were actually doing. On balance, my hand was probably better than a club, but only marginally better!

The everyday effort of life after the accident left me feeling constantly exhausted, but it wasn't as if I could afford to relax; there was still so much I had to work on. I didn't have the luxury of time to sit around vegetating. I had done that exceptionally well in my coma, after all! But no one else saw it like that; people would tell me I just had to be patient. So I told them, 'Patience is for people in hospital.' I knew

DOI: 10.4324/9781003244370-5

that just sitting around wasn't going to help my rehabilitation one bit, and I felt obliged to do every last little thing to put my body through its paces. I chopped up countless vegetables for my supper, just so I could practise using my left hand. I would never have called myself a vegan (or a kiddy-torturer, as I had sometimes been known to call them, tongue in cheek), but the routine of slicing, dicing, and chopping felt like good exercise, and I was trying to focus on food that might be helpful for my health too.

When I went out for a walk or a run, I held a sweatband in my left hand, just so I could practise moving it around and manipulating it in my palm, anything to engage different movements. I know! I sound like some sort of weird robot, being programmed to replicate human movements. But who in their right mind would have designed a robot like me?! Whoever it was had clearly forgotten a stand-by setting, because I was finding it impossible to relax knowing that there was something I could be doing – *anything* – to try to hasten my recovery.

In addition to relearning how to use my left hand, I had to learn how to use my right hand to write, eat, and do all the other things that would once have come so naturally to my left hand. Some of those changes are slightly easier to adjust to than others. It's fair to say that my occupational therapist taught me one of the most valuable post-injury lessons of all . . . how to get dressed! It may not sound like much, but until you've tried putting socks on when the world feels like it's falling away from you, or until you've tried to persuade a non-compliant arm into a shirt sleeve, you just don't know how difficult that is. The sheer bloody exertion involved in doing up my shirt buttons needs a chapter of its own! The OT did say that dressing oneself is one of the hardest things to learn how to do all over again.

I knew that it wasn't normal to keep myself on the go, every minute and every second of the day, every day. I knew

I needed someone to tell me to stop, pause, take it easy. But those soft words never came. My marriage with Liv ended, and that longing for someone to share my burden with went unfulfilled.

The signs that my marriage was ending had been there, I just hadn't noticed them. My chocolate oven glove of a brain could have made a goldfish look smart, so even when Liv was telling me or just dropping subtle hints that she was leaving me, I didn't pick up on them. And when I say 'subtle' I mean things like telling me she was buying a new house and suggesting that we should live separate lives until she was able to leave.

I was only dimly aware that when I was practising some simple movement on my own in the kitchen, my wife and children were gathering up all of their things to move into their new house. The excited whoops and laughter drifted through to me as I sat alone and silent.

The end, when it came, was long and protracted. I had to endure my wife and family leaving me in interminable stages, all in view of the scarers, and I couldn't adequately show them how I was feeling. My damn brain injury had seemingly left me incapable of looking like I could feel any true or real emotion. It seemed as though I was existing in a hinterland and witnessing the death of myself as a husband, as a father, and as a person, all while I appeared to regard it all dispassionately. I wish it had been otherwise; I wish I had been able to express how I was truly feeling. I wish that with one bound I had been able to cast off everything that compromised my status as a fully functioning human, but I was too broken in every respect. When she finally left, Liv wrote to say goodbye and said:

Never ever lose sight of the enormity of how far you've come. Those of us around you have been amazed to witness each victory however small on this marathon journey. And it really has been a marathon for us all. It's taken its toll on us in different ways. I will always be a friend to you and support you in your role as a father to our kids, but the accident robbed us both of a life we'd imagined and the marriage we had. We need to move on. You need to be the awesome dad that you are to your kids.

Reading that made me feel better and worse, but most of all, it hurt like hell. It only emphasised the strength of the bond we had once had. On reflection, I was pretty stupid to have ever thought things might have worked out differently. Perhaps it just proves the old adage that hope triumphs over adversity. Because I had never, ever given up hope that we would make it through the travails of life after everything that had happened.

Even after she was gone, I still harboured lingering hopes of getting back together with her. Life without Liv felt like another part of a puzzle that needed to be solved. Perhaps I thought that reconciling with her would have helped put the whole sorry saga firmly in the past. As if being back in that relationship, or even moving on and embarking on a new relationship, would have grounded me. Of all the things that you miss when a relationship breaks down, it is often the subtlest things you miss the most. I just wanted someone I could sit down and relax with, someone with whom I could enjoy the infinitesimally small victories, like when I beat my son or one of the scarers at chess.

But I didn't have any of that, and in the end, I just had to learn to let that spur me on too. Too many supposed experts had already written me off as a vegetable, and there was no way I was going to prove the buggers right. Not long after the accident, one of my colleagues had even told Liv that there was only a 30 percent chance of me ever being able to dress myself independently again. What a complete load of rubbish! Where on earth did he even get that statistic from? Actually, I think he got it from a place where the sun does not shine! The experts had all got one thing right enough, though: life was bloody hard work. So whenever I was struggling to do up the buttons on my shirt, I used my disgruntlement with experts and their statistics to spur me on.

It wasn't as if I had a choice. I knew I had to go on proving everyone wrong every day, but it only made me harder on myself. Whenever I got up from a chair in those days, my left leg was slow to kick in, and I would invariably topple over to my left side. I hated having no control over such rudimentary movements and knew I had to recognise the possibility of falling over so I could always be prepared to compensate. Apparently, it was rare that individuals took that kind of pre-emptive corrective action; people said I was unusual (but I hasten to add it was just one of many reasons why people said that about me!).

If nothing else, it did prove that I was still far from the finished article, as much as any Australian can ever be a finished article. Unless your definition extends to when I was lying – nearly dead – by the roadside in St Mawes; I was almost a finished article then, for sure. But where I saw all the imperfections and compromises, everyone else saw progress, and I was getting slightly sick of all the compliments I was receiving about my recovery. Yes, I was alive. Yes, I was better than I had been. But as far as I was concerned, my body was still buggered, and I wanted so much more than what I had.

Since my accident I had been surrounded by people who were paid to be around me, and people who were worried about me, and people who, for the most part, were telling me what they thought I wanted to hear. But I didn't want to hear how well I was doing; I wanted to be like any other adult getting on with his day without falling over when he got out of his bloody chair. I wanted to live a life where nobody had to see me walk through a doorway successfully and want to congratulate me for it. People told me it was remarkable just how far I'd come . . . well, I can tell you it didn't feel quite so remarkable when I was flat on my arse, having fallen over again.

Pragmatically I knew that I just had to do the best I could do with the hand I had been dealt. It was as simple and as stark a choice as: deal with it, or give up and die. Inevitably, there were times when I would have been far less emphatic about keeping on buggering on, but in many ways, I was too selfish to die. I wanted to go on seeing my kids, although I couldn't help but feel guilty about still hanging around the poor little buggers.

I recognised my own selfishness, but my desire to stick around must have been fuelled, in part, by my wife's less-than-emphatic answer when I asked her, 'Would it have been better for the family if I had died at the triathlon? Or if the doctors in ITU had turned off my ventilator?' What kind of question is that to have to ask your wife? I do understand that it must have been absolutely bloody awful for all of them, and especially Liv. A very good friend of mine, who also happened to be an ITU consultant, once told me that the doctors in Cornwall rang him to ask if he thought I would have wanted them to carry on treating me, as opposed to turning off my ventilator.

I know from my own experiences that turning off someone's ventilator is a little bit of guesswork, and you just hope that you get it right most of the time but also accept that if you do get it wrong, there is no way of proving that you got it wrong. Of course, the person involved is unaware of the situation – as I was – and they've got even less power to communicate their displeasure with your decision either way. In those situations, it all comes down to communication with the relatives, and you just have to try and help them accept that your decision was made with the needs of their loved one in mind.

I don't know what Liv went through, and we never did talk about it afterwards. Even though I was beginning to accept that the marriage boat had sailed without me on board, I often felt a very strong desire to be with Liv again. I still harboured that desire for reconciliation. As far as I was concerned, we had married for life, and I was desperately sorry that she saw the prospect of the rest of our lives together as a life sentence.

It wasn't just what we had lost that bothered me, I couldn't stop thinking about what we could have been and what we could still have done for our children. Of course I was 'happy' to have survived and to have been given a glimmer of another chance at life, but that didn't assuage all the guilt or the creeping feeling of knowing that I would never really be able to provide my kids with any useful coaching for playing rugby or tennis, or running. I know those sound like relatively minor concerns compared to the stark alternatives of living or dying, but I had never wanted to be stuck on the sidelines. I had spent too long watching my kids both metaphorically and literally racing away from me, while I just watched. At first, it was only sport, but as time went on, I had to learn to watch them grow up and race away with their normal lives too.

How do you deal with standing on the sidelines in your own marriage? Somehow, I was going to have to watch – and accept – that Liv would also race away into the sunset and another life. Liv and I were just more bricks in the head-injury wall. The experts didn't predict that, did they? They didn't tell me my marriage was going to fail as a result of my injury.

Am I saying, 'don't trust the experts'? Not quite. But I think a dose of healthy scepticism is always a good thing. How can someone tell you won't walk again? How can they tell you that you'll never be able to dress or eat without assistance? How can they ever say what you'll be capable of? I defied the experts; why can't you defy them too?

What is an expert anyway when their field is so poorly understood, and so little is known about how far one can recover? I do think all of us can make a difference to the body of knowledge on this subject. And with that greater knowledge comes greater hope for the future. The key to it all, for me at least, is determination and perseverance.

The sun was now well over the horizon, and the Falifornia day was heating up. Another run successfully completed – providing your definition of success amounts to keeping running feet in synch without falling over – I took an all-too-brief moment to feel proud of what I had achieved. . . .

I still hadn't achieved as much progress as I would have liked, and it hadn't been as fast as I would have wanted, but I *had* made progress, and I was *still* making progress. *That would have to do for now.* And for a while that was my mantra. My marriage was over, but I was slowly coming to terms with it. We had been so very strong on our wedding day, but we had been two very small people – Liv a relatively diminutive 5 foot 2, if you want to be precise – and we had been undone by a catastrophe we could never have foreseen. But I knew that we would remain good friends with a shared history that made us both happy. That, too, would have to do for now.

5 How Hard Work Helped My Mental Recovery Process

Life v2.0

One of the questions I was asked most often in my progression from Brussels sprout to appearing to be a relatively normal and independent adult was this:

'How have you managed to recover so far, so fast?'

It was a well-meaning enough question and almost always was intended to show some sense of commendation for my efforts. The problem was that I never felt able to give people the kind of answer they probably would have wanted. Objectively, the signs of recovery were there, of course, but I never thought or felt as if I had recovered that far; I still saw myself as a space-occupying lesion. To me – and perhaps to you – that was a big problem: if you get to a point where you can almost pass for the kind of person who hasn't just spent the last umpteen years of life in slow and painful recovery, how the hell does anyone know that there is anything less than 'normal' about you? Too advanced to be seen as having anything too seriously wrong with me and not capable enough to live the life I wanted, it seemed to me that I was just going to have to resign myself to marvellous mediocrity.

I was left wondering how long I was going have to sprint just to stand still. And there were plenty of days when it was difficult, if not impossible, to think that there could be a better life out there for me. Inevitably, there were days – too

DOI: 10.4324/9781003244370-6

many days – when I gave in to a little bit of unabashed, self-indulgent wrist-slitting. I hadn't died, but I did often feel as if I might as well have died. It wasn't some sort of suicidal ideation, more a case of *fuck it, this is not me! I am so much better than this bag of moroseness, this pessimistic waste of space*. It was easy to feel like that, sitting on my own, having lost my wife, my kids, and my occupation. I had woken up from my near-death experience, and the game had changed without me ever knowing the new rules.

But by Christ, I knew I was just going to have to make the best of it and carry on, because what else could I do except fall down and die? Fortunately, there were days – just a few at first – when I felt, if not confident, then hopeful for the future. And in spite of all my usual reservations, I could put a more objective spin on the question, 'How have you recovered?'

I knew that an enormous part of my recovery was down to my determination. Some people have even had the temerity to say I am stubborn! I prefer to think of it as being fully focused on recovering in the hope that there would be a better life out there. It wasn't all about me, of course. My wife and kids had helped in their own ways, both before and after divorce. And even when they didn't directly help, just the thought of them helped me stick to the course. Of course, my scarers were absolutely instrumental in helping me keep going too.

Whatever I did manage to achieve in my recovery – as well as whatever I'd managed to achieve in my life before the injury – I put down to hard work. That same dedication I had shown in my work-life definitely helped drive my journey towards a different life. I have always believed that most people who are successful in whatever they do have done a tremendous amount of work that nobody ever sees. So when golden opportunities present themselves, they are already best placed to reach out and grab them. I tried to exhibit that same attitude, knowing that every last little bit of effort I put into my recovery work would pay off in the end.

I was once told that what separates the wheat from the chaff is when and how you deal with adversity, and I suppose my recovery proved that. It's all well and good travelling along with your life laid out in front of you, navigating the occasional obstacles you put down for yourself whenever you do something ill-advised. But it's a damn sight harder when you have to navigate a bloody big obstacle slung in your path by some omniscient and omnipotent maleficent being! It felt like that's what had happened to me. That's what happens to all of us when, out of the blue, the cataclysm of a brain injury disrupts all our well-made plans for the future!

Being in some ways 'better' doesn't mean that we aren't still broken. And being given a second chance at life doesn't mean that we will always be sanguine about being so far removed from our previous life. My own iteration of Life v2.0 wasn't off to a flying start, and I was reminded, day by day, if not hour by hour, of all the things that were more difficult than they had been for Andrew-before-the-crash (or Andrew BC). If I had ever imagined that 'recovery' would progress in a smooth curve, then I would have been sorely disappointed. Incremental change and improvements did happen, but they didn't add up to a day-by-day sense of improvement. My burden didn't feel progressively lighter. Some days it felt heavier. And the better days were interspersed among long periods of torpor, anger, or sheer bloody frustration.

My journey from vegetable to near independence was hard to gauge objectively. There were times when all I could see were the years that had been taken from me and my family. And there were days when, no matter how well people said I was doing, I just didn't want to hear it. Besides, the course of that progress would have appeared very different from the outside, looking in. It was easy for people to see the improvements in my gait or my speech, but that didn't make up for all the time I'd lost not being able to play games with my children when they were growing up.

The problem is that people couldn't ever appreciate what my journey *felt* like. They equated progressive improvement with exponential gains in happiness, and it just didn't work like that. I'm very well aware that there were times when I came across like a selfish old bugger, seemingly oblivious to the progress I'd made, never happy with my lot in life and always striving for something better. I could have had an army of psychologists lining up to tell me about the deleterious effects that my less-than-perky attitude would have on my state of mind in the long term. Given how little of my brain was left, I suppose the fact that they could have spent any time pontificating about the state of my mental health was somewhat encouraging!

I realised of course – as everyone does eventually – that if you are going to try and make the best of your new circumstances, you are going to have to leave your old expectations behind, sooner or later. (For me it was later rather than sooner!) Objectively, 'moving on' makes sense, and in theory, it sounds fine. But you and I both know that the day-to-day reality of letting go is bloody hard. Every day, I felt weighed down with a world of loss and regret, with the added burden of a buggered body which never quite did what I wanted it to do.

The physical work of recovery was not always appreciably easier, but it did at least feel like a defined problem that could be fixed by hard work. One of the hardest things was relearning how to walk and run but in a way that went against my normal instincts for how to walk and run. I had got to the stage where I could play tennis reasonably well, and I could play various ball sports, but I still had a tremendously strong pull to the left, and people were telling me it was permanent; I'd just have to get used to it. That kind of talk was like a red rag to a bull as far as I was concerned. I'd had my fill of absolutes – you'll never have a fully functioning memory, you'll never walk unaided, you'll never do anything remotely human ever again – and I wasn't about to roll over and accept defeat.

While my bravado was all very well, it didn't help me ride my bike any better! In fact, I can safely say that riding a bike when you feel like you are eternally listing to the left and backwards was bloody well impossible. Depressingly, I knew that if it were not for the abnormal contraction of my muscles, I would have been able to cycle without any real problems.

Still, I wasn't going to be beaten, even if it meant doing something truly terrible. . . . I knew I was going to have to drum up the courage to ask one of my scarers to help me! It isn't nice knowing you need help to do something so simple that any reasonably coordinated five-year-old can do it, but it was at least better than the days when I'd had to have scarers standing by just so I could practise standing up safely. That had been really embarrassing.

Anyway, whoever it was who said you never forget how to ride a bike can take a running jump! As well as all the other experts, I had managed to prove them wrong too. It took a lot of work, and it was accompanied by an awful lot of loud, incendiary vocalisations, and yes, that's the polite way of telling you I swore at the problem like a good Australian should. But bit by bit, I got steadier and more secure, and I proved a few more bloody experts wrong. By God, it helps to have the fire of righteous indignation to keep you on track to any goal, and it certainly spurred me on countless times.

And so it was that as I sailed (relatively) smoothly down the road like a kid leaving his father and his stabilisers in his wake, I ruefully reflected on the state of my life as it was then: I had been forced to deal with living life as a Brussels sprout; with losing my vocation, which I had loved; and even with seeing my wife and children leave me . . . but at least I could ride a bike! Small comforts.

I hadn't even stopped to worry about getting back on a bike, given that the whole sorry adventure had begun after being knocked off my bike in the first place. But I was pleased that there was no need for a further unplanned intervention from the Cornish ambulance service. How different things would have been if it hadn't been for them. And how different things would have been without my friends. There is no doubt that my friends and carers did so much to help me along my journey. Even now, not a single day goes by when I do not count myself lucky for each and every one of them. Not just my friends from before the accident, but my scarers, who were so resolutely patient with me at every tentative footfall and with every tortuous revolution of a wheel around its axis as I swayed, swerved, and wobbled towards my next achievement.

I had always thought that a life well-lived would be a fairly linear process, in which one is continually moving forwards in all things. And one of the cast-iron signs of living well would be never spending too much time looking backwards, but always focusing on the here and now, with one eye on the future. A bit like cycling, then! And in pursuance of the metaphor, I was determined to concentrate in the here-and-now of getting myself better and look to the future with an eye on striving to reach my previous physical state.

Realistically, though, I knew that it would be exceptionally difficult for me to ever get remotely near to my previous physical state. As if I did not have enough reminders of how bad I was, well, my cycling was just so awful and precarious, even when cycling around the back streets of Falifornia. On the plus side, at least I had a partially metallic head, and what with my helmet, too, I felt pretty sure that any car would come out of a collision worse than I would!

If there is any danger in looking too far ahead, then it is surely in reaching that point in one's thoughts of the future when, inevitably, one is not around anymore. In the depths of my darkest depression, I had seen that point in time and had even thought of conducting my own eulogy. In thinking of it, I perceived that I was considered as being quite a nice bloke, possessed of loads of very good friends, who were all so instrumental in helping me to continue, and crucially, kept giving me even more reasons to keep going. It got me to wondering about the chicken and egg argument: was it me that had shaped my friends in some way, or did my friends shape me into the person I had become, the person they all wanted to help? I'll gladly take a significant part of the credit for being able to bring out the best in that band of reprobates, of course. Likewise, I'll take some credit for being able to even recognise they do have some positive attributes that didn't come from their associations with me! Don't worry, they'll all know that I'm messing with them, and perhaps that's important too. . . . I needed to be able to maintain the same kinds of relationships I had always had with those people. I needed to be able to be just as forthright, rude, and contentious as I ever had been. I needed, in short, to go on being me, and they understood that.

So I'm not going to try and claim that I am solely responsible for all of my goodly attributes. (Perhaps I put in one too many o's into that word, 'goodly', but I will leave you to work that one out!) And neither am I going to try to claim that all my faults lie with them, not even when my mood slipped and every little thing made me angry.

My sister was running late because she had a meeting? Angry. My scarer failed to overtake a slow driver in the car? Angry. My supper did not turn out well, or my cafe still didn't have the cake that I loved? Really angry! I know. I *know*! First-world problems, right? But what do you do when literally everything makes you angry? How does anyone cope with that?

Even though I recognised that feeling angry was a totally inappropriate response, it still got me down because I had never been that way before. And even though I knew it was a pointless waste of energy, I found it so hard to shake those feelings, even though, in every single case, I was the one who ended up suffering. Because I had been so used to being a relentlessly happy person, the change left me with a low-grade feeling of self-loathing. The stark dualism of my human nature astonished me, and through it all, my friends remained to help pull me through to the other side.

Howsoever my friends found me and however I ended up in their lives, I knew I was lucky to have them, and I felt so beholden to all of them – including many strangers – who I relied upon to help me in so many significant and insignificant ways. The woman at the reception area at the local hotel pool who had always had a kind word and smile for me never knew how important she was. The vivacious woman at Tesco's at Pendennis Point (or what you might be able to guess I call Penis Point) who told me she had enjoyed my writing.

Inevitably, thinking about the paths my life had taken as it intersected in and out of my friends' lives made me think about Liv and the children. And it was some time before it occurred to me that I had never properly grieved for the loss of my wife and my family. Later, I met someone whom I felt would have been perfect for me, but she told me in no uncertain terms that she was not interested. Even though I knew it was only that one person I had lost, I couldn't help but pour the feelings that I should have had for Liv onto her rejection. I'm quite sure that Freud and his band of psychologists would have had a field day with that, just as I'm sure there's a perfect multisyllable word for describing it. But in the wake of it, I felt Liv's loss more keenly, even more so than I had felt it when we separated. The hurt that I had probably been denying all that time hit home, hard.

You'll be glad to hear I didn't ever let my decorum slip, though. I still felt a sense of obligation to try and remain upbeat for all of the people who helped me and the people whose lives crossed into mine on a daily basis, like the woman at the reception desk. Because every smile from every stranger mattered. Just as those friends who didn't change who they were when they saw how much I had changed also made a difference. So, to go back to that chicken and egg question, I suppose we are the product of our surroundings and the people who surround us. The fact that, in the early days after the accident, Liv travelled the two hours every day just so that I could go on seeing the children, so that we could still feel as if we were a part of each other's lives, mattered. It made a difference.

6 How I Learned to Live A Life of Compromise After Brain Injury

Life in Falifornia!

I think I may be preaching to the choir when I say that one of the hardest hurdles for me to overcome in my recovery was wondering:

Am I to be defined forever by one mistake?

And the answer was equally inescapable and depressing.

Whatever my life was going to look like, it was going to have very little in common with the life I'd loved before. In every way.

It seemed unavoidable that my new life would only ever be a life built around struggle. From the very start, I felt as if I was fighting so hard, just to ensure my family would not be as adversely affected by that one calamitous mistake as I had been. I was already removed from their lives, and it sometimes felt impossible to accept that. How do you make that transition from being a happy, healthy, fully functioning family to being torn apart? How can you ever accept it when the blame isn't in your relationship, it's in some bloody, near-fatal quirk of fate? Yes, couples grow apart, and relationships break down. But for very different reasons. How do you ever live with knowing – pretty bloody certainly – that if it hadn't been for that one mistake, your own family would have survived and prospered?

DOI: 10.4324/9781003244370-7

Feeling so removed from my children's lives, and of any chances of ever being able lie back with their mother and talk about all the little things that make up one's life with children, felt just as crippling as the accident. We would never while away the time talking about how they were doing in school, or which university they were going to attend, or who they were dating. We would never have the shared joy of becoming grandparents. We would never be there for each other, never support each other through illness or deaths in the family or our own old age together. . . .

When I reflected on what I would have wanted to be happy, I didn't ever feel as if I was asking for too much. I only ever wanted what I had already had. Nothing more. And that seemed especially unfair. Someone once told me I'd been given a unique opportunity to reinvent myself. It was the sort of opportunity that some people dreamed of, but I can assure you, it was an opportunity I would never have asked for.

I wrestled with the question of work. Wondering if I could or should re-train, but everything felt so far removed from anything I had ever done before. And I still felt so inept and ill-equipped to do anything meaningful or anything helpful to my future. I was surely too old to start again. I hadn't been able to accept the end of my family, and I couldn't accept the loss of my vocation either: knowing that I would never again do the job I had loved. Mentally, I kept finding myself drawn back there, imaging that I was still capable of doing what I had done before. Daydreaming that I was still turning up at my allotted time, helping so many people, taking a good wage, and then going home to my 2.5 children and my wife. They were the things that kept me awake at night.

But then, on a good day, I'd counter all of the misery with thinking about how lucky I was to still be living in Falifornia. It wasn't all doom and gloom; there were times when every bright sunny day in Falifornia felt brighter and better than the last. I knew my worldview must have seemed slightly schizophrenic or perhaps, more correctly, bipolar. I knew that I had to cherish the positive days. I had to try to make the most of every opportunity and each bit of help I was offered. And help was never less than abundant; whether that was because of who I was or who I had once been, I didn't know.

As my journey into the new life I hadn't ordered continued, I was amazed at the number of incredibly brave people I met, and it made me completely reappraise my definition of bravery. Any survivor of a serious head injury is an absolute walking miracle, a true testament to perseverance, motivation, and unwavering courage. Liv had said that to me, and it bears repeating to you now.

From meeting so many people who have not only survived but prospered in the face of adversity, I think that it is not what one has had to contend with that makes a person brave, it is acknowledging our fears and facing up to them. Just being able to get up the next day and the next and put on a sunny disposition is bravery in action. It reminded me of the English question I was given in school, to compare and contrast the bravery of two characters in two books. One of them was a priest in a Graham Greene novel, who was constantly questioning his vocation, and the other was a priest who blindly followed his religious beliefs, even though he knew it would lead to his execution. (In other words, his blind faith put him on a fast track to sitting with the Lord a little sooner than he would have planned!) The answer was obvious to me then, and it was comforting to know that my opinion hadn't changed at all. I knew bravery when I saw it.

That didn't mean I knew how to be brave, of course, I just had a damn good stab at it. I acknowledged my good days when they came along, even some great days. There were days when the Falifornia sun shone, and I went for a run, followed by a swim. I'd have coffee and cake in my favourite café and then meet some friends on the beach. Those were objectively good days, but even then, I couldn't always shake that lingering feeling of being useless and rudderless.

I was still so paranoid of being just another sad, lonely, divorced bloke with nothing to distinguish me from anyone else in the same parlous situation, and I'm fully aware of how arrogant that made me sound. But why should there have been anything to distinguish me? My God, living life after the crash was a lesson in self-actualisation, and I wasn't always sure that I was up to living by myself. I felt like such a boring, pointless old fart. I thought about the homeless people I saw sleeping rough around Falmouth, and I couldn't always say there was any real difference between them and me. It just happened that I had a house and a shaver and a mirror. I used to see some of those men and women out busking; that would have been absolutely out of the question for me – I was completely tone deaf.

I felt that I had lost so much of just being able to sit down and be content – not ecstatic – just content. (I had almost certainly given up on ever feeling ecstatic again.) But ecstasy's more straightlaced cousin, contentment, was just as elusive. When it came, it was fleeting. And I wondered if that lack of contentment was one of the root causes of my general unhappiness.

In a way, I felt selfish. The amazing efforts of the NHS and all of the committed people who work in it had, in essence, resurrected me. But it seemed to me that all I had been doing was thinking about myself and my recovery to the exclusion of everything else. I was in the midst of my own existential conundrum, and the feeling that I needed a higher purpose and to be achieving some greater good wouldn't leave me alone.

Rudderless. That's how I felt. Cast adrift on an ocean of self-doubt and uselessness, and still a bit lopsided to boot! And as if that wasn't bad enough, there was another issue that was becoming increasingly clear to me. And for an Australian, this one had the potential to be even more damaging. . . .

I was starting to feel more and more like a sensitive, soppy sod. I had gone from being tough on the outside, tough on the inside, and impervious to excess sentimentality – or to put it another way, Australian – to being sensitive about anything and everything. I had started to see hidden meaning in everything, even the most unlikely things. For example, if I saw a van drive past advertising a business from an area where my old hospital was, it made me think of my old life, the life I had just thrown away. Or it could have been an old couple walking by, arm in arm, looking effortlessly happy in each other's company, and it would make me think of everything I had lost. Any time I took the children to the cinema, something would inevitably set me off too.

One evening, I watched *Mamma Mia* with my daughter, and all I could think about was how I had thrown my life away. It was supposed to be a nice occasion, something 'normal,' but I suppose that was what made it feel so abnormal. It's hard to make the adjustment when you are supposed to feel grateful because you can do something as simple as watching a film with your daughter. In that moment, I knew that I didn't have anyone else to think of in life, other than myself. As much as my kids were – and remain – so, so important to me, I couldn't feel as if trying to give them an evening of simple entertainment was enough for me.

One day we watched a film with a cartoon animal who was crying out for his mummy, and all I wanted was for my kids to call out for me, but I knew they never would. They would only ever call out for their mum, because what would I have been able to do to help them?

I didn't feel it in a 'woe-is-me' kind of way, well, perhaps a bit, but more than that, I was just so aware of having to embark on an entirely new life, without ever having wanted that life, and being saddled with more issues than Germaine

Greer fighting for feminism. And the cumulative effect of all the emotion was to impress upon me that I needed to be occupied all of the time. The more I dug down into it, the more I understood the depressing existential reality that I was just so bored with myself. But I was stuck with myself too.

There were of course many reasons why I had turned into such a bloody bore; chiefly, I was still grieving for my past life. But knowing that didn't bring any comfort. Knowing why you're unhappy isn't necessarily going to shake you out of feeling unhappy, and it seemed to me to be bloody unhelpful when I was in the midst of dealing with it all. It felt a bit like being trapped and drowning in a sinking ship and knowing that there are other people who are also trapped. Thankfully, I've never been in that position, but I can only assume it's not exactly helpful knowing that other people are drowning while you're drowning!

More than that, I was tired of the constant drudgery of my new life, and I just couldn't see myself ever doing anything productive again. I did appreciate that, in many respects, my life was objectively better than it had been following the accident. I even had a routine that incorporated my daily activities with my exercises. On most days, I got up in the morning – unsurprisingly enough – and had a shower. Now, at this point, I should say that I do not intend to give you a full anatomical rundown of my washing procedure, but firstly, I scrubbed my hair thoroughly, then I had to reach for my flannel on the small shelf in the shower. But I did that with my eyes closed, meaning that I had to try and differentiate the flannel from the various soaps and other paraphernalia I had accumulated. I did that with my eyes closed to try and improve my proprioception; I had had to work hard at regaining any sense of feeling and acuity in my hand and fingers, so the daily scrabble around for the flannel, which never seemed to be in quite the same place two days running, was a decent workout. Then I would try to stretch up and touch the ceiling with my left arm. For a long time after the crash, I had been unable to lift my elbow above the horizontal, back when it was little more than a useless club.

I should say at this point – in case my mother is still reading – that I always made sure to check that the shower mat was securely affixed to the floor, or else I would have run the risk of looking like an elephant dancing on ice. It's important that people know you're being sensible. 'Sensible!' There's another word I hate. I mean, who in their right mind (or their wrong mind, as in my case) would want that on their tombstone? *Here lies an incredibly sensible man.*

Anyway, having very sensibly done the main part of my ablutions, I would then brush my teeth, which, of course, I did standing on one leg. I looked a bit like the can-can dancers, as I kicked up one leg at a time to practise my balance. I have to say that the ice figure-skating champions, Torville and Deane, had absolutely nothing to worry about from my less-than-elegant movements. Then I used my electric shaver and attempted to shake the living daylights out of the endolymph sloshing about in the semi-circular canals in my middle ear – or to put it more correctly, I did my vestibulo-ocular exercises. The fluid in my ear was causing all of my wavy perceptual problems and making me feel sick and unsteady to boot.

My balance remained one of my most significant issues, so I had to spend large parts of the morning making myself almost sick with dizziness, as I shook my head back and forth, whilst looking at a fixed spot on the wall. These vestibulo-ocular exercises were designed to help me equilibrate my brain with the actual world, as opposed to the one that I was perceiving, and as such, I used to believe the vertical was 30 degrees to the left. All of which helps to explain why I was always listing slightly to the left! It felt like there was a magnetic force pulling me that way.

So, after all of that exertion, I was invariably ready for coffee. It's fair to say that my coffee consumption had reached stratospheric levels, but again, it was easy to blame my determination for that! Everything that went with brewing my coffee was on my left, so it gave me lots of practise using my left arm and hand.

The final act in ensuring I was ready for the day was bending down to put on my smart shoes. Never mind the fact that I was absolutely terrible at walking in them, at least they gave me an opportunity to practise tying my shoelaces again – and who doesn't want to have to re-learn that most basic skill decades after perfecting it the first time?! And so, dressed up to the nines, or perhaps just dressed up to the sevens, I walked into town and rewarded myself with a fantastic coffee – it must have been at least an hour since my last one – and a piece of cake in one of Falifornia's numerous cafes. Combining exercise and activity was a way of trying to re-learn simple multi-tasking activities. During the day, I always tried to cram in some more balance and trunk-strengthening exercises and worked on my writing and on my memory. And at night, I got back into can-can mode to brush my teeth.

It wasn't a terrible way to live in reduced circumstances, but it was the same every day, and increasingly, I realised that while I was superficially enjoying myself, it really was only superficial. Such was the regularity of my day that I was getting bored with my life. There was no greater purpose to it, and I felt like I was capable of more. I must have been the fittest cripple in the park, and yes, I was repeatedly told that I needed to stop calling myself a cripple, but I would say that it is only ever me that I'm describing like that. And only because one night I went to bed a married man with a family, a career, and a body that was pretty bloody good at endurance sports, and then came back to existence in a hospital bed, crippled, unable to walk or use my left arm. Like most Australians, I'm far too used to calling a spade a spade, and if something is not working 100 percent then it is buggered or worse. I am certainly a product of my upbringing, and in the eighties, at an all-boys school in Australia, terms like that and others to describe anyone who was not as sporty as the rest were unfortunately used quite liberally. So I ask you to please indulge me and remember that I am using that term here in a positively negative way.

Nonetheless, lots of people happily told me (as if they should know) that my self-confidence should be sky-high because of everything I'd achieved to get to where I was. They meant well, but all I could think of was the endless parade of low moments that happened with monotonous regularity. The months and months that I'd had to be supervised getting out of a bloody chair. Assuming you have never suffered a head trauma, just imagine for a moment what it does to your confidence when, as a fully grown adult, you get into trouble if you try and stand up without first asking a carer for permission. And if that doesn't feel too bad, you can add in the fact of your spouse and your children leaving you and losing your vocation too, and see how that makes you feel.

I wasn't sure I should be believing the buggers anyway. It was all very good them praising me to the skies, but I didn't want – or rather, I couldn't afford – to get complacent. Not for a second. And so I focussed inwards and concentrated on making incrementally tiny but important improvements every day. And I can tell you exactly what that was like. . . .

I saw kids walking around town with far too much hair gel on, their locks gelled to solid peaks of perfection. Turd polish, I called it. You know that expression 'you can't polish a turd'? Well, that is exactly what I felt I was doing. Never mind the hair, I was just trying to polish the turd that was my life.

7 How Trauma Makes Us Reinvent Ourselves

Surviving Death by a Thousand Cuts

If working towards some semblance of physical recovery had been hard, putting back the pieces of the life I had once had was even harder. It felt like I had endured death by a thousand cuts, and life – what was left of it – felt like it was slipping away. I just didn't want to slip into oblivion with it. I hated not having any opportunity to discover anything new, waking up each morning or going to bed each evening just hoping the next day would bring some novelty. I liked eating cake in my favourite café, but I didn't want that to be the high point of every day of the rest of my life. Even when some days were better than others, they didn't bring happiness. I knew by then, if I hadn't known it before, that happiness was much more than the absence of sadness.

The remedy? Because I was just so damn bored with myself, I knew I needed new things to focus on. I kept coming back to the idea of work and wondering what I could possibly do to feel useful. I realised that my job had been a huge part of what had given me my sense of self-worth, and without it, I was bored and boring. I had always loved my work; it really had given me everything that I could ever have wanted. I had been providing useful help to people who had needed it, and I had a degree of respect by dint of what I was doing. It had been intellectually stimulating, and there had been a teaching element which I loved. I had relished being part of a team of like-minded individuals; we all

DOI: 10.4324/9781003244370-8

worked together for people who needed our help. I used to get home tired at the end of every day, but it was a good kind of tired, not like the feeling of exhaustion that had been so present during those endless days of struggle through rehab.

I missed helping people, I missed my former team, and I missed using my damn bowl-of-porridge head for something remotely useful, as opposed to just baiting my scarers. I know that my scarers would have found me contentious and argumentative at times, but as I said to one of them, I was merely testing the veracity of their belief. I loved pitting my wits against others, and it was an important part of who I had been and who I still wanted to be. I think it was important for me to be able to try and identify what I perceived to be the various strengths and weaknesses in the people I met, and in my scarers, so that I could use their strength of conviction to challenge mine. (And yes, I did actually say that some of my scarers had strengths. They know that I loved them, really!)

So I recognised the need to challenge those parts of my personality that had been deprived for so long. In doing so, I hoped that I might find some sense of purpose. I think that the yearning for a role in life was one of the strongest in my personality. One's sense of purpose is a combination of parts, both external (where someone else gives you a sense of achieving something, like getting a medal in a sport) and internal (like those feelings one gets when one has run a very good race and knows there was nothing else one could have given). Or, to rephrase that in the context of my old working life, I had been used to the external validation of gratitude from people I had helped and the internal satisfaction of completing a task well.

I knew I needed to find my role and satisfy my sense of purpose, otherwise I would have felt like I had been salvaged and done all that rehab work for nothing! Aristotle knew what he was talking about. His philosophy of virtue is still so very relevant for the 21st century. He said that we need what he called telic and atelic activities in our lives. Today, we would understand that to mean goals (telic) and activities that we do without fanfare, purely because they are enjoyable and/or worthwhile (atelic). Atelic activities usually have no end point, but they often provide opportunities for growth and, to coin the hip phrase of the day, well-being.

I didn't have enough of either. It may sound like a stretch, but I felt like a stroppy teenager, who, having missed two kicks at goal, gives his football boots an accusatory stare as he throws them to the ground in a fit of pique. But it wasn't my boots I was annoyed at, it was of course my buggered body that was deserving of my derision. (Fortunately, it would have taken a feat of supreme physical flexibility, far beyond my ability, to have thrown myself to the ground. So I was at least spared the indignity of throwing myself onto and picking myself up off the floor!)

To put it another way, I felt like I had just graduated with a generic degree, not really equipped to do anything. I had gone from having a working life with a career path and a ladder to being forced into retirement. (I should say that I have many friends who have taken voluntary retirement, but unlike me, they hadn't been forced into it.) It brought back a memory of my mother asking me if I was ever in a position where I didn't have a job and could not get one, would I consider the army. I am not sure, but I think my ambivalence towards authority was relatively obvious even then. Her seemingly innocuous question brought on floods of tears, and I told her that I would rather be a criminal than join the army. In my young mind, I couldn't get past the idea that the government's need for a police force and a judiciary showed a tacit acceptance that their rules were not going to be followed anyway. So it made no sense to me. I was already seeing the world as a series of contradictions and wondering where I was going to fit in and make some sense of it all. But none of that helped me when now, decades later, I would wake up at four in the morning paranoid that my life was not going anywhere. I was told it was perfectly normal for everyone to experience that kind of ennui, but I had never experienced anything like it before.

I knew of course that it is not normal to be happy all the time, even under the best circumstances, let alone when you have been smashed into by a car and are piecing your life back together. (Not even a truckload of Prozac can achieve that level of happiness.) But neither is it normal to wake up petrified of the day ahead because one does not have any plan beyond the same three or four things every bloody day. And that was the question I kept being asked: what is your plan for the day? Every time someone asked it, it just seemed to highlight my failure to find anything useful to do. It felt depressingly like I had come to the end of my useful life.

The brand-new life that I had been given came with so many impediments that I have forgotten to even tell you about all of them. Plenty of specialists drifted in and out of my orbit, ranging from a neuropsychologist to a podiatrist (their primary job, though, was to help me deal with the loss of sensation in my left foot). I don't remember much of my work with the neuropsychologist, but I can tell you that my feet have been very well looked after! I also saw a behavioural optometrist to help with my hemianopia (a partial loss of sight after the accident). They prescribed some prism lenses initially, and I now use special glasses to help me compensate for the lack of a complete visual field.

But you probably won't be surprised to hear that, of all the problems I've forgotten to tell you about, one of the largest impediments was my memory! I couldn't always recall what I had been like or how easy I had found my life before the accident, but of course, it had seemed fundamentally better in every way. I hadn't ever woken in the early hours, worrying about my life and where it was going. Back then, I just used to get up, get out, and set about my day. But I also remembered how Liv had told me that I was too used to thinking of my life as Andrew BC with rose-tinted glasses. I started to wonder if she had a point.

I thought about my friends and their lives. While I had always been quite interested in what they were up to, I realised that I had become much more inquisitive about what my friends were thinking and feeling. That was an interesting development, and sure enough, a positive one. I started to feel like an anthropologist, actively observing how they lived their lives, as well as trying to observe my own life with a little more objectivity, and in the process, I found that many of my thoughts felt quite new to me. In particular, there were all-new feelings of anxiety. If I had to go out and socialise or meet new people, I found it extremely tiring and anxiety-inducing. The tiredness was at least partly because I still had all of that lingering doubt about my body's ability to keep holding me up, so that when I prepared to stand, I had to ensure that I kept my left knee slightly bent, rather than locked straight, or I would have been at risk of staggering or falling as I rose to my feet.

It may sound like a ridiculous metaphor, but balance really was the elephant in the room. (Perhaps my subconscious was trying to tell me something about the weight I'd put on and worked so hard to shift after the crash.) But my balance was so variable, and because it was so fundamental to doing anything like a normal-looking person, it tended to loom large when I did anything at all involving other people. You can't underestimate the impact of having all of those doubts and all of that abstract worry in the back of your mind, even when you're just talking to people. So of course it was tiring.

I found that I needed a rest day after being sociable, even though, on the surface, I hadn't done anything more taxing than eating and drinking with friends. That wasn't like Andrew BC. But increasingly, I was having to try and accept that I was not that man that I kept referring back to anymore.

I would have described my old self as being quirky, kind, and generous, possibly even a bit hyperactive (although not in an ADHD kind of way). He was optimistic and appreciative of things too. So much of that was gone, and some of it would never come back. My template of who I was had been rewritten, and my neurons were still so buggered that I didn't quite know if I'd amount to anything ever again.

Buggered but bouncing back? Fucked but still fighting? They were the questions that I kept on asking myself. . . .

It's hard to judge just how you're doing in the middle of an existential crisis. But there were plenty of times when I would have given you just four letters to make a suitable word describing my mental state. Perhaps if it had been a game of Scrabble, I'd have given you a six-letter word to make an adjective in the past tense. By this point I had had six hard years of fighting back, not so much a life as a life sentence. After all of that time, I was less fucked, but I was most definitely still fighting for every tiny improvement. The question lingered: *how long am I going to have to fight?*

One of the things they don't tell you about starting all over again: it's a hell of a lot harder when you're older. It's hard to have to learn about all the things you can't do, such as walking down the street and talking on a mobile phone at the same time, or using a knife and fork whilst eating, or writing anything more legible than a spider dipped in ink and running across a page. It was all a far cry from being able to turn my hand to almost anything, as I had used to be able to do.

I was feeling increasingly paranoid about getting older still, knowing that I had so much less time in which to start over. I was so far off being a fresh-faced twenty-something, and I had dependents. The time when I could just get pissed, have a laugh, and live without any real consequences was past. While I had made a lot of new friends, including my many scarers, and while I had made scraps of progress, there was never an end in sight. I was still making for that same bloody finishing line that I had set out for all those years ago.

People sometimes described me as being endlessly negative or maudlin, but I would have argued back that I was exceedingly upbeat for someone who had almost died and lost everything that had any meaning to him. Anyway, I was not a complete idiot, and in view of everything that had happened to me, I was not about to go running through the tulips in the manner of Julie Andrews, singing songs about raindrops on kittens or some variation on 'isn't life grand?' Admittedly, that is partly because I am tone deaf. In fact, an old girlfriend of mine had the temerity to say that I even hummed in a tone-deaf manner! So, I wasn't always being negative; most of the time I was being willfully self-deprecating. That was a big part of the positive-negative attitude that had taken me that far and kept me committing to the search for something better.

Once I'd argued people out of thinking I was too negative they would often change tack and try to tell me that everyone's life changes as they move through it. My own life, they ventured, was just going through some changes too. But I had to disabuse them of that notion. For most people, if they're lucky, life changes come in small steps, giving them time to adjust to new opportunities or, in my case, new constraints. There were no subtle degrees of change for me; I was instantaneously resurrected into the form of limping mental cripple. There I go again calling myself a cripple. And there I go again with the self-deprecation. But my frustration was all too real. My memory was a good example of how that change manifested itself. I used to have an effing superb memory for facts and random information, and the frustration of just losing that overnight was stupefyingly embarrassing. In time, and with considerable effort, my memory did improve, but I had to put my chocolate oven glove of a brain through some extraordinary workouts to get it going again.

When things went well, or I was able to acknowledge some little scrap of progress, I did allow myself a nanosecond of excitement that perhaps I was starting on the threshold of a new path. I just had to stop comparing the horizon that lay in front of me with the view of the verdant grasslands I'd left behind. Even if/when you reach a point where it looks as if you're all set up to start again, it's hard to get past your sense of what life used to be like. That in itself is quite ironic; given the ease with which I managed to lose so many of my memories at the time of my accident, I never lost that sense of just how much better my life had been. But knowing that I had to find a path with some degree of purpose in it meant having to suck it all up and bloody well go for it. I didn't know if I was setting out on a brave new world or destined to remain flailing about on an ocean of regrets and self-flagellation, but not knowing wasn't going to stop me. That's the positive-negative spirit in action!

The work on my memory – on *everything* – did at least point to my unwavering determination to revive some sort of life for myself. I didn't want to slowly atrophy into a life of insignificance, I wanted to leave my Brussels sprout years behind. Just as I desperately wanted to be self-sufficient, and to do all of the things I needed to be able to do in life without having to rely on others. I hated having to depend on carers from 8 am to 8 pm every bloody day.

More than anything, I wanted to be able to help people in a meaningful way, take a decent salary, and work in a team for a predefined, set goal. My friends tried to find work for me, but they thought I needed to do something menial; they didn't appreciate what else I might have been capable of. Of course, they were all very well-meaning, and they all wanted the best for me, but I knew that I was capable of so much more. Andrew BC had had it so good, and I didn't want a lesser life. So it was difficult feeling as if I had to prove myself to everyone all over again, only this time it seemed like an utterly intractable process. Despite my limitations and my complaints about my reduced capability, I did not feel as if I had collapsed so far backwards, just that I was starting from a very low ebb. In some ways I felt as if I could have done almost everything that I could have done before, but I was overlooking something. . . .

Before I could find work or do very much else, I had to engage in the much harder work of trying to learn what it was to be me and what I still needed to do to become a fully independent adult. On the one hand, you could say that I had left what you might call 'my previous life' in a surgical bucket, but I still felt as if, in a way, Andrew BC's life and all of his experiences were still there, somewhere, amongst all of that surgical detritus. I was effectively a new person, and I was still working out what that meant, but I didn't subscribe to the idea that I had lost access to the old me entirely. I felt as if I still had access to the keys to my brain, I just couldn't quite locate them. And that's a thought I'll come back to in the last chapter. . . .

Practically, though, everything that I took as normal about my life, I had to re-learn. Even such simple things as remembering to pick up my keys before I left a restaurant, or remembering to wait before everyone was seated and then waiting until the ladies had started eating before I could eat. As well as all those relatively prosaic things, I had also had to re-learn that one needs to constantly work backwards, such as when driving anywhere, one needs to plan when one wants to arrive, and then work out how long it will take to get there, as opposed to just setting off and arriving, as if by magic, at the right time. Or, when putting on clothes, one has to start by putting on the clothes that are going to be removed last. 'Pretty bloody obvious, you idiot,' I can hear you say, but it seemed like a revelation to me that in so many ways, we live our lives backwards. And perhaps that helped reinforce the sense in me that, although I didn't know what I wanted to do in my life, I knew what I wanted it to feel like. That was the end point, I just had to work backwards to find out what job or pursuit would provide that feeling.

I was still somebody who judged my own self-worth by what I could do for my family and those I loved, as well as for anybody that I had the power to help. I had always been a doer, I had always felt compelled to help whenever I went anywhere, as if I had to be seen to be contributing. But over the course of my slow recovery, I learned that, sometimes, you can just sit in the presence of your friends and not really say a lot, not really do a lot, and still participate, still contribute something even without consciously trying to. That was something of a revelation to me. And in that, I came to understand that helping people could take other paths. . . .

I started to think about retraining to become a life coach. It seemed like it would be the fastest way for me to begin helping people again, and I rather arrogantly thought that being an associate professor in medical ethics and law, coupled with my medical background, would stand me in pretty good stead. And oh yes, there was the small matter of my recent life experience too.

A funeral helped put some things in perspective. They do that, don't they?

It was the funeral of the local parish priest, and it led me to consider many of the similarities between what I did in medicine and the role of the parish priest, as well as the 'misrepresentation' of 21st-century medicine. I worked in intensive care, a setting of immense emotional stress for patients and relatives and, not infrequently, for staff as well. Intensive care can appear more like the cockpit of an aeroplane – full of machines that bleep and flash as they keep patients alive. This, however, can belie the true meaning of what we do. There is an evolving misinterpretation of what medicine is:

that 'good' medicine in the 21st century is skill-based technical wizardry, where 'good' doctors are people who can diagnose, treat, and cure using magnetic resonance imaging (MRI's), gene therapy, or laser-guided scalpels and the like. I believe that what a patient wants, first and foremost, is a physician who is compassionate, honest, and committed to their cause. Without these underpinning attributes, their drive to find the best treatment for each of their patients will be diminished. William Osler said in 1907 that 'You (physicians) are in this profession as a calling, not as a business, as a calling which exacts from you at every turn self-sacrifice, devotion, love and tenderness to your fellow-men. Once you get down to a purely business level, your influence is gone.'[1] And for *'business level'* one could insert 'disease or diagnosis'. The patient is just one part of the whole person, just as the successful treatment is just one part of an illness journey (albeit a vital part). Knowing the physician is compassionate, committed, and honest forms the foundation upon which the scientific wizardry starts to work. It also has a very real beneficial treatment effect (the placebo). And this is where Aristotle returns to the fray of modern medicine.

Aristotle's *Nicomachean Ethics* sets out the three stages of virtue ethics: *arête* (knowledge), *phronesis* (practical wisdom), and *eudaimonia* (flourishing – performing as an expert).[2] Part of knowledge is an understanding of what personal attributes (dispositions such as compassion, humility, justice, and courage, which Aristotle called 'virtues') are required to 'flourish'. As doctors (and I assume clergy) become more knowledgeable and experienced, the good virtues (dispositions) that make them strive to do the best for patients become ingrained in their performance. Put generally, we professionals – sailors, gardeners, mothers, etc. – have a duty to do what we do with good intentions. And the more we do this, the better our abilities will be. Andre Comte-Sponville has said that to flourish is an individual's accountable task; virtue and especially compassion are pre-requisites, and to be without them is to be 'inhumane.'[3] Virtue is 'a force that has or can have an effect': it gives the person their distinctive excellence. It is this acting well that makes a person 'more humane'. In Immanuel Kant's terms, it is one of the individual's duties to others.[4]

An Aristotelian 'good doctor' or 'good priest' will not always make a good decision. Indeed, there is a circular argument here: it could be considered morally presumptuous to assume a consultant physician is virtuous, or good doctor just, on the basis of training or level of seniority, and therefore that they will always make good decisions. But this in part misses the point. It is the underlying virtues of a doctor that will make them reflect and study and, coupled with experience and a desire to determine what is in the patient's best interests, that will lead to good decisions. Put more simply, it is the underlying virtue to help that is necessary to start being of help.

I wanted to be of help. I had identified that need in me. Perhaps I didn't even need to be a good doctor to do that. I had a lot to think about. . . .

Notes

1 Osler W. The reserves of life. *St Marys Hospital Gazette*. 1907; 13: 95–8.

2 *The ethics of Aristotle: the Nicomachean ethics* (translated JAK Thompson, revised Hugh Tredennick). London: Penguin Books, 1976.

3 Compte-Sponville A. A Short Treatise on the Great Virtues. London: Vintage, 2003.

4 Ameriks K. 'Immanuel Kant', in *The Cambridge Dictionary of Philosophy*. Ed. R. Audi. Cambridge: Cambridge University Press, 1999.

8 How I Proved That Almost Anything Is Possible After Brain Injury

Advantage Tillyard!

I can't remember much of what I was thinking about as I was being voluntarily electrocuted and forced to crawl through a slurry pit, but there was probably a burgeoning sense of achievement under the pain! Five years after the accident, I was taking part in a Tough Mudder event. In case you don't know, they're the sorts of challenges people take on when normal marathons seem a bit too staid and safe.

I had a team to help me, of course. I couldn't have done it without them, and I am eternally grateful to them for enabling me to put my body through the kind of test I simply couldn't have imagined in the earliest days of Andrew AD. I may have lost a lot of weight since the earliest days of my recovery, but I still needed help climbing over a 20-foot wall. I did suggest they just throw me over, but even I had to admit to being too heavy to be used as a javelin. So my team ensured that I completed the course unscathed, and for that, I was immensely grateful, given that, at the time, I still found walking down the street without falling over challenging enough. To complete a Tough Mudder was a whole new level of achievement, and stratospherically greater than anything that could reasonably have been expected of me.

It's true to say that I probably wasn't reflecting on the enormity of my achievement as I was wading neck-deep through the slurry pit and crawling agonisingly slowly under the electrified fence, where every wrong move sent shockwaves

DOI: 10.4324/9781003244370-9

running through my body. Then there was the small matter of a 60-degree hill to run up. . . . Who says I don't know how to enjoy myself?!

Emboldened by my success, I sought more challenges. On the surface, going to Australia felt like no kind of challenge at all. It was certainly diametrically opposed to the challenge of a Tough Mudder. I had been on a plane to and from Australia many times before the accident. But practically, it proved challenging enough. I think some people worried that I might somehow get lost on the plane. Even with my limited understanding it seemed to me that it is not really possible to get lost in an object travelling at 30,000 feet with no doors to escape from.

It seemed to me that while the Tough Mudder was designed to prove I could be left to my own devices, the trip to Australia had been designed to show me how I could not be left to do anything independently. And it's hard to try and live in the moment when you have a squad of scarers primed to step in and talk you out of whatever it is you want to do that contravenes various health and safety regulations! I didn't like that at all, especially in the land of Burke and Wills. . . .

A little Australian history for you: Burke and Wills were two famous explorers who went on an ill-fated exploration through the middle of Australia. From the outset it sounded completely unachievable, if not ridiculous, but it was inspiring too. Whenever a good friend and I came up with some suggestion for hijinks or an ill-fated idea of our own – usually involving beer and a longish trip through a municipal park or an ever-so-slightly-precarious walk along a cliff face towards a beach party – we relied on our mantra:

'Did Burke and Wills say why?'

'No, they said, "why not?"!'

There was something in that indefatigable approach to life's problems that (obviously) resonated with me. I was facing similarly insurmountable odds to get my life back on track, indeed to just survive. And I did not want to be restricted by asking myself 'why' when I could be asking 'why not?'

That was the kind of thinking that led me to compete – unaided – in a half marathon a couple of years later. I would never have imagined that it would have taken me quite so long to get to the point of being able to run 13 miles, but at least I didn't think it was going to take me that long to finish the bloody thing! (In fact, I was told that I would need a digital stopwatch to time myself, as opposed to a sun dial!)

While Falifornia isn't exactly renowned for its flat, savannah-like wide open planes, its steep, steep hills made it seem more like the Grand Canyon to me. I could already picture the scene: the breathless marathon runner – excuse me, half-marathon runner – tumbling down a hill and being shoved in an oxygen tent by a paramedic. For some reason, my scenario was weirdly embellished to show the paramedic smoking as he put me in the rarefied atmosphere of the oxygen-rich tent and then the two of us going up in a blaze of smoke.

There had definitely been times when the thought of going out like that – in a small-scale, makes-the-local-news kind of blaze of glory – might have appealed. I don't think it will surprise any of you to know that. But whenever I found myself wishing for the exit door, it was rarely, if ever, in any way that could have realistically happened.

Even without the threat of explosion, I found myself at odds with my care team, who did not think I should have been competing in anything other than a brisk walk to the shops and back. I thought they would have known me much better by then. If they had, then they would certainly have known that their reservations were like the reddest rag to the surliest bull.

The event itself was quite routine, and I neither exploded nor disgraced myself, so I suppose the most interesting thing about the whole incident was the way in which it demonstrated how I was feeling about my injuries at the remove of seven years. When you're in recovery, people tell you how you must appreciate the severity and significance of the injuries you have had. How you need to think in term of the long-term impact, not a quick fix. I didn't want to – or couldn't – accept the even harsher reality that the effects wouldn't just be long-lasting, as I'd been told, but life-lasting. I was always far too much of an obstreperous old bugger to accept that.

I felt like I had experienced too many examples of my body winning the battle of will versus action, whenever rehabilitation had seemed too hard or whenever my legs failed to do what I expected of them, and I had always had a ready excuse: my brain was damaged! What else did I expect? But I never quite knew if the root of my issues with coordination and movement occurred because my body was sending such divergent signals to my brain or because the brain was interpreting the signals incorrectly. It was like a yoga teacher saying, 'You need to listen to your body,' only to hear that the body was sending back all sorts of erroneous messages.

I always thought that my experiences would be a fertile ground for philosophers or anyone interested in existentialism, and in reflective moments, I tried to do my own existential investigation. While I felt too stupid to give precise, unambiguous words to what I meant, I thought about what was left of me.

What is a human life anyway? Can it be reduced to wistful contemplation? Because that is how Andrew AD had spent so much of his time after the accident. I did not die, and although I am pretty certain there are no such things as ghosts – well, certainly not ones that can type – I sometimes felt a bit like a spectre at the feast. There were times when I felt as if all I had left were my memories.

When I started to tell the story of my incredible transformation from brainless Brussels sprout to whatever kind of autonomous vegetable I am now, it didn't just bring it all back to me, it made me relive some of those things. And I had to confront the fact that I really had lost everything that was dear to me. It didn't matter how many times I typed out that I had lost my wife, my family, and my career, it never lessened the impact of those things, not one little bit.

Not everything that I had lost was completely removed from me, but life felt so far removed from what I ever thought it would be. In the time it took for me to be knocked off my bike, everything changed. (And if it feels like I'm coming back to that one moment time and time again, it's because – as you may well know – you never really leave it.) All that was left of my relationship with Liv was my wistful contemplation of times past. It was a bit like bathing in the starshine of distant stars when you know that those stars are already long since dead.

I couldn't help but think that all we are in the end is our memories of times past. I supposed that I'd had the marvellous opportunity to experience death and a second coming, albeit without the beard and the walking on water. But it hadn't just been me going through that process. All of my friends and loved ones had experienced my near death and had to confront their own memories of what had been. To think about who I was and who they had effectively lost.

I continued to believe that, in spite of everything that had been taken away from me, my personality had remained more or less intact. My brain, for all of the damage it had suffered, had retained enough of my memories and experiences that continued to inform my actions and reactions to events. And I reasoned that if my brain had sufficient capacity and was still in full control, then the full, unfettered, uncensored Andrew Tillyard would remain a viable and hopefully vibrant presence in the world.

So much of my BC personality had been predicated on my relentless levels of activity – some may have been tempted to call it a preposterous level of activity or even hyperactivity – but as I have mentioned, I was able to capitalise on that element of my personality to my advantage in my recovery. It helped spur me on to try to achieve something new almost every day and then – and here's the scientific bit – flog it to death! It was the flogging it to death part that helped consolidate new learning and new movements.

Think of an undamaged brain as being a bit like a packet of uncooked spaghetti, where each piece of spaghetti is equivalent to a neuron. In an undamaged brain, each neuron runs in parallel and connects up appropriately to the next one in a series. This enables communication with the effectors, the organs or cells that respond to stimuli, which in this case are the muscles. When your packet of spaghetti – or rather, your brain – is in good shape, it is an easy process to transmit a command to the muscles. The moment you think of an action, the transmission process is so seamless, you feel that movement in your muscles almost instantaneously.

But a damaged brain is rather more like a bowl of cooked spaghetti. In this case, each piece of spaghetti is randomly thrown into the bowl. Transmitting an action communication to the muscles now needs to go across so many other neurons (or pieces of spaghetti) prior to reaching the effectors, and it is all too easy for the transmission to get lost somewhere along the way. But, as I found out, you can still work with a bowl of cooked spaghetti. You can still make sense of that jumbled-up brain, and all you have to do is practise. Over and over again. The more an action is practised, the more consistently you will activate the correct neuronal pathways and activate the effectors.

At around that time, I was also taking martial arts lessons. As with so many aspects of my recovery, it was mostly about balance. You could argue that it was as much about achieving some sort of psychological balance, but the martial arts training was all about the physical. If you're reading this wondering if this was the start of my journey to black-belt proficiency, then I'm afraid I'm going to have to disabuse you of the fanciful notion. I'm not even sure I'd have been capable of landing a head kick on the most diminutive of Snow White's seven friends! Nevertheless, the work did help solidify my balance and did wonders for my speed and movement, particularly on my left side.

But at that stage in my recovery, I was reflecting on the fact that, from day one, I had been told that, at some stage, the gains that I made would start to tail off. And seven years in, I didn't want that to happen. I refused to let it happen, in fact. I was quite happy that I was still making improvements. I had actually managed to halve the time it took me to do my regular run, and while there weren't any metrics or measurements that I could use to compare my balance, the instructor was certainly impressed with the improvements I made.

It tallied with my belief that the neuronal pathways which were there prior to my accident – back when I was still Andrew BC – were still there. It followed, therefore, that *all* I needed to do was to provide the neurons with the correct stimulus to open them up again. I did believe that I could, at least partially, get back to where I had been before. In a way, I bloody well had to believe it. What other option was there? Anything less than that would have felt too depressing. And if I thought that my body could recover, then I also wanted to believe that of my cognitive ability, including my memory and my clarity of thinking. They had been there before, I just felt as if I needed to ensure the correct stimulus to ensure they could be 'resuscitated' too.

But memory is a funny thing, isn't it? It's incredible, really, that we do not really know precisely what memory is or how it works. Is memory just a neurotransmitter, i.e. a chemical that makes a neuron fire in our brain? Well, one way to answer this question would be to compare the brains of a series of trained and untrained animals to assess the biochemical difference. By 'trained' in this context, I mean an animal that has learnt a do a new task, akin to Pavlov's dogs slavering over the sound of a bell. It could be rats who are adept at following and then seemingly remembering a certain path in a wooden maze.

What happens in our brain when we try to remember the *Mona Lisa*? Is the image like a series of pixels? Like a digital photograph in our head? Is the number or pattern of neurons that fire when we remember it the same ones that fired when we first looked at the actual painting? Do we have to think about the image in order to turn on the pattern and trigger the appropriate neurons? That's all well and good, but could that also work for non-visual memory? Could there be an analogous situation for the neurons that deal with auditory memory or smell? And what would direct the neuronal firing to the visual memory cortex, as opposed to the auditory memory cortex?

And what happens if you can't remember? Perhaps we need to reframe the problem; perhaps the issue isn't with our memory at all. Perhaps the problem is with recall.

It's fascinating that what we perceive is everything to us, such as in that old question: if a tree falls in the woods and no one is around to hear it, does it make a sound? We are so bound by what we believe we know to be true, even if the truth is flawed. If I think about what I was like initially after the accident: I thought the vertical was angled 15–30 degrees to the left, which is why I always leaned to the left and why I always fell over to the left. Quite quickly, I had to reappraise my understanding of the vertical; well, I had quite a lot of incentive to do that anyway. And so, with a lot of embarrassment and hard work and persistence, or stubbornness or focus or whatever one wants to call it, you can make the brain re-learn these things. Even a bowl-of-porridge brain like mine (or a bowl-of-spaghetti brain) could do it with the right kind of stimulus.

So it was that sort of thing that got me thinking about that question of whether what we perceive is just whatever the brain is telling us. Take an incredibly vivid dream where we feel as if we are actually living the part that we have designed for ourselves, so that we can feel as if we are parachuting through the air, and we swear that we can actually feel the air rustling though our hair, and for all the world, it feels completely real.

That was what my dreams were like when I was recovering from my injury, and I could swear I was playing tennis and feeling the sun hot on my back, and I could hear the tennis ball hit the middle of the racquet and feel the characteristic feeling of a fine shot as it pinged off the strings. Thwack and bounce on the line. And when I think about it even now, that feeling of the hot sun on my back still stands out so much. How is it that we can feel things that are not actually happening to us? It's like virtual reality (VR). If it is quite as potent and as powerful as that, why wouldn't one want to get the latest in VR technology and go on a virtual holiday? I can answer that one: just think what will happen to humanity when we all decide that, rather than pay an exorbitant fee to a travel agent, we're going to stay at home in our VR headsets!

All of which thought and speculation brought me back to the big question: why is it that when you have had a brain injury, you cannot simply reboot? Like turning the computer off and on again. And if it's true, as I pondered earlier, that all we really are in the end is our memories, then surely it's how we choose to interpret these memories that makes us the people we are. Or, to put it another way, we are each like books in a library. Despite the fact that every word has been used and there are really no unique words, the order of the words is unique in every person's story, and that's what differentiates each book. So if we really are a product of our memory and our perceived experiences, can't we just tap into those and reset ourselves on the right track?

My vivid dreams had certainly given me a taste of the life I wanted to lead, and by the time I had turned limping into relatively fluid walking, I was able to blithely go about my day, pretty much able to do most things to some degree of competence. But let's be honest, they were no great feats of athleticism, usually walking and running to my next piece of cake! Somehow, I was expected to be happy with that, and of course, I wanted more. For me, outside of my dreams, and lacking a VR headset, tennis was the hardest nut to crack.

When I started trying to play tennis again, it seemed to target all of my weak points. To say that my left arm still didn't have a lot of sensation in it was putting it mildly; it couldn't have fought its way out of a wet paper bag. And when I say it didn't have 'a lot' of sensation, you can read that as practically no sensation. I think I should rather say that I could barely feel the bugger at all. (And that's why, when I ate with a knife and fork, I needed to put on a wetsuit first because of all the mess I made, which was sadly ironic given how often I used to tell my kids off for eating like a pride of lions at a trough.)

Then there was my balance, and you know the routine by now . . . when I say I did not have great balance when I started trying to play tennis, you can read that as no discernible balance. If I needed to walk across a room with a mug of coffee, I would almost invariably end up going on a trip to the plastic surgeons with third-degree burns! Whenever I tried to move quickly and to change direction from the way I was moving to hit a ball, my left knee locked up straight, so I was left trying to move quickly with a 'Jake the peg leg' in such a manner that it lacked any degree of finesse (as much as any Australian can be described as having any degree of finesse!).

And lastly, as if that litany of issues was not enough, there was my vision. If we'd played with tennis balls that were the size of beach balls, I might have had a better chance of hitting the damn things. But as it was, I seemed to have lost all ability to work out where the ball was in relation to myself. I could follow the ball to my left and to my right, but I couldn't seem to work out how far away it was from me in three dimensions. And so I was left waving my racquet around like a fly swatter aimed at an elusive fly. I couldn't even work out which side of my body the ball was going to be on. To sum up, then, there was my useless left arm, a complete lack of balance and vision, and a brain that felt like it was constantly rebooting. The likes of Andy Murray and Pat Cash had nothing to fear from me!

But the exact same rules applied to practising tennis as to everything else. It was just that with so many different elements to work on, it was a bit of a slog. I had to break the game down into its many component parts, then work on the simplest elements and practise them ad infinitum. It really was as basic as just bouncing a ball in front of me to try to catch it again so I could establish where a ball was in relation to me and respond accordingly.

It helped, of course, that I was a very hard task master. I was more ambivalent about the fact that I had always found tennis so easy in the past, and now it seemed horribly, frustratingly, impossibly difficult. On the one hand, I was really trying so very hard to not get too down about struggling to recapture just some of what I had lost, while on the other, I was hanging onto the vision of hopefully being able to do it again. But my goodness, I had to work at it! And of course I got frustrated, and of course people couldn't understand why. It was only because I needed to do so much hard work that I carried on saying my body was still rubbish or broken. And what they could see was a former cripple – my words, not theirs – trying to play tennis, trying to challenge himself again. How inspiring! But what they couldn't see – or feel – was the impact of all of my muscles fighting against me. It may have looked like a struggle to hit that bloody ball, but they couldn't have understood that it had been a fight to live for so many years prior to me even picking up a racquet again.

At some point we all have to take that next step from merely existing, post-injury, to living. I was pretty sure that I'd got the existence bit down pat, but I didn't want to just exist, I wanted more. So I was determined that, in that stilted cooperation between brain and body, the brain would come out victorious. I wanted to turn *Deuce* into *Advantage: Brain!* I wanted to move from who I was into who I could still be, who I wanted to be.

Much like me, the tennis did improve, and it is still improving, but the work was like a full-time job in itself. There were days when I needed to think of the work of recovery like that. I grew to love my morning routine of a run and then a swim. Even now, it still sets me up for the whole day and makes me feel alive. And perhaps that is one of the benefits of recovery . . . when the normal, everyday movements that you learn in childhood are taken away from you and you have to develop whole new ways of doing things, you experience some different responses to them. Or at least you notice them in a different way. Now when I swim and I feel at one with the water, it is a joyful experience. Perhaps even more joyful than it would have felt before the accident. It certainly helped my worries and cares melt away. Of course, the worries and cares were all still waiting for me in the changing room with my trousers, but having a break from them could make them feel a bit more manageable.

I think I can trace my indefatigability back, long before the accident, to my mother, who instilled in all of her children a real drive to better ourselves. Thanks to her, I carried that 'never say die' attitude. So did my sister. By all accounts, she was literally yelling at me when I was in my coma in the intensive care unit! So, even without consciously registering it, I was propelled through recovery believing unambiguously that, so long as there is a pulse, then there is a chance. A chance to do something or achieve something, however big or small.

People say, 'it is what it is. . . .' That would be anathema to Mum, or equivalent to swearing. Dad gave my mum the platform upon which she could drive herself to perfection or drive everyone else to distraction; they were a great support team. And so, waking up from a coma with that kind of insurmountable determination, I could only ever have survived. The experts said I had almost no hope or prospect of recovery; what did they know? With no malice at all, I have been known to refer to experts in neurology as experts in levitating. They might just as well be for all we know about the brain and its remarkable ability to recover.

I started out trying to find common ground between the brain and the body, between my cooked and uncooked spaghetti, and I did, in time, find the whole me. And now you're stuck with me!

9 How to Go on Living A Life of Value After Trauma

It Takes a Village

Right from the start of my emergence, blinking, into the world of recovery, I was told – or at least my family was – that I would not be able to summarise anything, or assimilate information, or distinguish the main point from a paragraph or a set of information. And neither would I be able to retain information long enough to do any of those things. So that put reading off the agenda.

Reading had always been such an automatic pleasure in life, but the power to read anything was lost to me. There I was – a bloody doctor – and I could not even read a sodding kid's book. It was because of my homonymous hemianopia, which meant that each line of a book was left overlying the line below it. That was coupled with my left-sided issues which also meant that I missed the first part, or the left-hand side, of each word. So if I was reading about a pancake in a giant picture book font, I would be left wondering why the person was flipping a cake.

For God's sake, I couldn't even read a picture book to my kids! Lateral thinking took me so far, and in the early days, I literally had to work at memorising each page of a picture book in order to 'read' to my kids. The irony of it was that while I was doing that, I was giving my kids 50p pieces for each book they read, all while I was unable to read anything myself.

My God, the lengths I went to in trying to compensate for my not seeing the beginning of each word. I even tried a

DOI: 10.4324/9781003244370-10

computer programme that would convert any text into one I could more easily read. It highlighted the first letter of each word in red, but it wasn't a long-term solution. Then there was the most enormous and cumbersome device made for me by the physio, which allowed me to read each line by itself, which stopped the overlapping line issue. It helped, but again, I wasn't going to blend in very convincingly on the train with one of those!

The vision was one problem. The memory was still a bigger problem. There are of course limits to what any of us can remember, and I felt as if I was routinely pushing the limits of mine. It's all too easy for a man who has left half of his brain by the roadside or in the surgical bucket of detritus to forget where he has put his glasses. Again. Or where he has put his latest drink, even when it is on the table in front of me. Don't even get me started on trying to find a parked car in a car park! We are such visual creatures, and ordinarily when we walk through our living room, we can just scan the room for our wallet and keys. And if we have just left them behind, then, when we see them, they become a visual prompt, a handy little memory backup. So, without fully functioning eyesight or short-term memory, my efforts at reading were off to a pretty bloody terrible start!

They were very dark days indeed, but I pretty much vowed to myself that I had to be able to read again, I just had to. So I was soon fighting against those preconceptions of who I was and who I could be. I knew that my brain had created those pathways and neurological connections in the past; it was just that, in my revised state, my brain was essentially a blank canvas of old, broken roads and pathways running between numerous towns and cities like Assimilation Town and Summary City. I was left trying to excavate them and build them anew. Not for the first time, I felt like an archaeologist, trying to find some sense of the future by working through the wreckage of the past.

It was difficult work. Overcoming these sorts of issues is the sort of work that goes unnoticed – and unconsidered – by most people. And for far too long, for so much of my time in recovery, I was stuck with just my own dark, dark thoughts to occupy me because I was unable to read a book or even a newspaper. Being left to stew in your own thoughts is hard enough at the best of times, and it really isn't very healthy being stuck in your own head with only your own thoughts for company when you have had to endure the loss of your wife and kids. But like an enormous, fat cow chewing the cud, I was used to smiling and masticating, trying to look pleased with my lot for the benefit of the people around me. At times, I felt an unbearable pressure to be upbeat for all of my scarers. You may agree that one of the greatest difficulties of living life in forcibly reduced circumstances such as this is in appearing to be one thing, i.e. happy, when you are anything but happy!

So I worked on my reading and I worked on my short-term memory. My mum would set me five words to try and remember each day, and just like building up any other muscle, I managed to build up my memory to the point where it was able to remember five random words, then eight random words, which as she freely admits is more than my mother can do!

The work paid off, because when one word of a book led (relatively) seamlessly into another, and then one paragraph led inexorably into the next, my world opened up. I felt as if I had escaped! I was finally reading a book, and I had left the cage of my prison far behind. I know this is not exactly revolutionary – depending on the choice of book, perhaps – but nonetheless, it was a very significant moment for me to get some relief from my confinement. It's interesting to note that 'confinement' is the same term used by women when they are pregnant. It was pretty much the exact opposite with me in that, rather than producing something beautiful at the end of it, I was just working on another version of myself. I was pretty confident that I wasn't going to emerge as pretty and perky as a new-born baby.

Trying to read lying down in bed was a different proposition. Everything I had learned to do to facilitate my reading when sitting upright went slightly skewed at an angle, and it introduced too much complexity to reading each line. That being said, as soon as I had identified the challenge, I needed to prove to myself that I could read sitting, standing, or lying at any bloody angle I felt like! One tenet of my recovery was there's no going backwards, and by God, I was up for putting that mantra to the test.

The first book I picked up and actually felt able to carry on reading was *A Short History of Nearly Everything* by Bill Bryson. (Feel free to file my book next to his when you've read it; I'm sure he wouldn't mind.) The introduction felt like it was written just for me and seemed almost unbearably meaningful. (Then again, I was feeling very sensitive at the time.) It talks about how tenuous our hold on life is and how real change of our species takes a millennium. Reading that, all I could think was how I had taken the one life I had been given and completely ruined it, despite its promising start. Just reflecting on that redoubled my enthusiasm for making sure my life did not impact my kids in any deleterious way. I hoped still that I could, in some way, give back to them some of what I felt my parents had given to me.

That sense of continuity and of giving back had gained extra importance to me. Throughout my journey back, and in this book, I had reflected on the impact that my scarers, friends, and family had made and thought about our mutual reliance on each other in so many areas of life. I'm sure Mr Bryson would have had a few things to say on that score too. The moments that we share with others to get us through our day are some of the most important, undervalued interactions we have. And it was that shared sense of teamwork, of responsibility with my wife that I really missed the most.

We still met up for lunch, but they were bitter-sweet occasions, and I'm not talking about the menu. Both metaphorically and literally, I felt like old news. A bit like: *so you had a crash and came off your bike, what have you done since then, eh?* On one occasion, Liv asked me if I would ever give up on my search for a job or for some meaning in my new life, and I wasn't able to answer her in any cogent way that would have satisfied her or set my own mind at peace. She knew, better than anyone, how my life had been so very much defined by my job, my vocation. The job was me, in more ways than I would have cared to mention. There was a new me emerging, but it was still consumed with all the memories of what was and the reflections of what could have been or *should* have been. I just needed to find a path that successfully combined the past and the compromised present into an acceptable future. Easy, right?

Plenty of people told me I just needed to belt up, stop living in the past, and stop going on about everything that had happened. It seemed like there was an expectation that I would resume my rightful place as the life and soul of life's party. At least, that's how I remembered Andrew BC, even if another friend did say to me, 'Don't worry about that, you were never the life and soul of any party!' So I suppose that gave me one less thing to worry about. I'm pretty certain that he didn't know the old adage 'don't kick a man when he's down,' but having said that, it was a miracle the man who said it could walk and chew gum at the same time!

I placed real value in looking forwards, but at the same time, I was conscious of how one's history can't help but predicate one's future, or at least one's reactions and responses to the future. I knew my past couldn't help but hold me back, and I had to find a way for it to drive me forwards, while ensuring my travails did not impact too much on my children. I knew that I had been a huge anchor on my family and friends, and I had never wanted that. (I hadn't wanted to have to manage without them either, but that's another issue.)

The problem is that, for many of us, there is no such thing as living *through* the trauma. What happens, year by year, is that you start living *with* the trauma. It can feel like a long, interminable continuance of a life, in isolation from family and friends. Some of us are lucky: good friends stay close by; good jobs stay open and available. But not everyone is so lucky. With neither family nor job to accompany me into the next phase of my life, I had to find new reasons for carrying on. I quickly came to the conclusion that needing to feel like I had to start again wasn't enough, I had to *want* to start again. But of course, I just wanted someone to be able to share it all with too.

So much in life really is dependent on effective teamwork. The president of a company or country is really just the figurehead to a team that is working flat out in the background. It is this shared responsibility you enter into with a marriage. You may or may not have identical goals, but each member of the team can recognise when someone is heading off-track and bring them back to the light, as it were. It is this shared responsibility that I missed so much. Like presents, it is almost always so much better to give than receive in any good relationship. Not that I was equating my new life as being some sort of present, unless it was a joke present given by a friend who loves to play practical jokes! I had always known that things are so much better when they're shared. But my children had not had that level of contribution from me. And it hurt knowing how many years they had been denied an active, present father.

They had had to contend with my loss, and likewise, I'd had to contend with their loss. So much of my identity went with them. Working as a doctor had been almost everything to me, it was my essence; I loved feeling that I was of some help to someone. People even used to call me 'selfless,' but I think I could have coped with the loss of my career if I had had my family there to support me. Just knowing that I had them would have helped preserve so much more of my fragile sense of self.

How easy it is to fixate on oneself when there is no one else to live for. How hard it is to carry on with all of the onerous recovery work you have to do when there is no one to support you. I felt as if I was so lacking without my significant other, without someone to share the day-to-day wins and losses.

I feel as if I had always been conscious of the need of support networks in our lives, but living a life of what you might call familial deprivation really rammed that home. I couldn't help but focus inwards. My single-minded focus on getting back some semblance of my life had been so all-consuming that I felt I had become every bit as boring as I had once feared.

It seemed to me that I was just like water. Certainly not because there was anything pure or clear or unambiguous about me, but rather because there was nothing interesting or intoxicating about me. As a plumber once said to me, when you have a leak, the water will always find the easiest way to get out. In the early days, weeks, and years after the accident, I felt as I lived in my bubble of being a cripple, limited to activities that were unspontaneous. I had used to be able to spontaneously play football or tennis, and I had even been quite coordinated and sporty – the first choice in the school line-up for the sports teams. But in the early days of my rehabilitation, I lived my life just doing whatever was easiest for me and not doing anything different in the way of exercise.

As time wore on, I became increasingly keen that, when I did anything with my children, they could see me engaging in it positively and with some measure of competence. My son told me how much he was looking forward to seeing me so that we could go for a run together. He seemed desperate to do it – not as desperate as I was to do well when running with him, though. I knew it was wrong, but I couldn't wait to (hopefully) beat him again too. My God, he was just 12 years old at the time, and I was 'desperate' to beat him. I knew that couldn't be right on any level, but in my defence, I will say that he did at least seem to enjoy the competition between us. It had only been a few years since he and his sisters had been pushing me around in my wheelchair. That's a lifetime for many arachnids and some small mammals!

*

Socrates said the unexamined life was not worth living, and I can tell him for absolutely nothing that the constantly re-examined life is not much cop either. I wanted my field of dreams, but all I actually had was a barren patch of land, bordered by some decidedly hazy and sketchy memories.

When I was told that my old job was not the same anymore, I regretfully came to the conclusion that not only was it not for me but that I didn't actually want to do it anymore anyway. I still wanted to do something that gave me a sense of achievement.

I thought a lot about what it is to be meaningful and useful, and I kept coming back to the same question: can intelligence be taught or learned? Bear with me here, as you will see how this one question inevitably gave me the answer I had been searching for. . . .

If I had ever had to teach a class in intelligence, I would have had the benefit of my own experience of having to re-learn virtually everything. And, based on that, I would have started my course with teaching the importance of sceptical inquisitiveness. Lesson two would obviously ask the question: what's the difference between humans and bacteria? What bacteria do by dividing some more to become a different or more resistant order of bacteria, we do by written word and communication. In other words, the greatest human invention is not the wheel or the engine; it is writing – having a technique of passing down information to the next generation, what we have learned. We want to help people in this generation so that they can move on, or progress forwards without having to make the same mistakes we have made.

And so, reader, I started writing a blog and then this book. (I told you I'd get to the punchline eventually.) Writing gave me a focus beyond my own horizons. It gave me some sort of purpose beyond simply doing my own thing for my own benefit day after day after day. And as people got engaged in my story, my life did start to open out more. I actually started to get requests for advice. Imagine that! People wanted to hear what I had to say about the experiences I'd had. Strangers got in touch to say thank you. Somehow, at last, I had found a way to help people.

10 How to Find True Love and Happiness After Brain Injury?

The Rule of Thirds

I was booked in to see a GP I had not seen before, and I was somewhat surprised, if not embarrassed, when he described me as being a bit of a hero. I did not really feel that I was doing anything special other than simply existing, and sure, there was a time when that was a truly amazing feat. So I replied that, while I was of course tremendously grateful for his compliment, there really was nothing heroic in managing to go to the loo by myself. Let's not even get into the business end of the whole business of going to the toilet! Just getting into position and getting trousers on and off was a supreme act of balancing, only made possible if I had a wall on my left-hand side just in case I lost my balance. So really, with all apologies to my GP, that was sometimes all I really felt like celebrating, albeit cheekily.

So I didn't feel particularly heroic, and I was really only dealing with the hand I had been given and trying to find a way of carrying on while appearing to be as 'normal' as possible. While the days when the chances of completing a successful trip to the toilet were less than 50-50 are now, thankfully, long gone, so too are the days when I could play – and even excel at – Aussie-rules football. And that was the point, really. There were still so many things I couldn't do that it was hard to celebrate some of the very rudimentary things I could do.

DOI: 10.4324/9781003244370-11

Over the course of my ongoing recovery, I had had to find ways to function which were completely new to me, i.e. ones that I had never had to do before to achieve whatever simple thing I was trying to achieve. Messaging and emailing friends had become a major undertaking. Instead of just rattling off a message and hitting 'send' I now (still) have to painstakingly ensure I have spelt every word out in full and that I have not missed out the beginnings of words. I even need to send any messages I write on my phone to myself so that I can read them and check them on my desktop before I send them. Then, and only then, can I relax sufficiently to send them out to the incredibly lucky recipient!

Of course, I understood the inextricable link between exercise and fostering better physical and mental well-being. During exercise, muscles, fat cells, and the liver release a variety of molecules into the bloodstream. Some of these molecules circulate through the body, where they can cross the blood-brain barrier. Once inside, they trigger a cascade of beneficial changes that can make one feel sharper and happier: one crucial change is the release of a growth hormone called brain-derived neurotrophic factor, or BDNF. When it comes to exercise's positive effects on the brain, BDNF is the foremost part of that process.

There is always the chicken-and-egg argument propounded by those couch potatoes, i.e., is it the exercise per se that is beneficial, or is it just the mere fact of doing something that one enjoys that leads to the improvements in mood and memory? Our brains are like a spider's web of connections, with links between different parts of the web, and these links allow the brain to combine the positive action of exercise with the positive effects on our brains and the BDNF that strengthens these connections, hence the 'runner's high'. And the more one practises using these connections, the more strongly they are formed or held. Doing exercise and practising the executive functions of the brain go hand in hand.

Otherwise, it can feel a bit like trying to grow grass without any fertiliser, and in this analogy, the BDNF is equivalent to the fertiliser. To take that analogy a step further, if we want there to be a very good covering of grass next to our house, then we need to ensure we put a lot of seed there, just as if we want to ensure our memory retains its clarity, then we need to go on using it and stretching it.

I am almost proof positive that massive improvements can be achieved. My slate had essentially been wiped clean (although the cleanliness of my slate may have to be considered under review). But having been wiped clean, I worked hard to start filling it back up again.

I think there are more important elements at play in my slow journey from vegetable to passing-for-human status. The first – and for better or worse it was something I feel as if I was born with – was my control freakery! It may be that it will help you to develop a bit of this too. (At least you'll be able to say, 'I may be a bit of a control freak, but at least I don't have an Australian accent!')

Take my obsession with running, for example. When I was finally able to ditch the training wheels of attendant scarers and start to run on my own, I hardly stopped. Was it any wonder that I became so obsessed with running when, at the time, it was the only aspect of my life that I had sole control over? Think about the typical aspects of life that one has control over: a career, a significant relationship, a family. . . . I felt as if I had ceded all control in those areas to someone else. But my running? That was mine. How much and how little running I did, how far I ran, it was all solely dependent on me.

As well as my control freakery to spur me on, I had my dogged determination. I had always thought that other people in a similar situation following a similarly life-changing event would, sooner or later, respond in the same way. But I remember when a chap in the swimming pool remarked on what progress I'd made. I hardly even knew him, but he had indirectly seen the improvements I'd made and said that I needed to keep up all of my exercises that I had undoubtedly been doing. And then he said, 'I don't think many people would have come so far with their recovery.'

My mother had been a nurse, and yet she had still retained her unfailing practicality and good common sense. And she surprised me one day by agreeing that it was surely my dogged determination that had propelled me so far in my recovery. Actually, I prefer the word 'focussed' because 'determined' has an ever-so-slight sense of the pejorative about it.

But if you aren't 'blessed' with the control freak gene and if you haven't yet found that streak of dogged determination (or focus), there's something else that can supercharge your progress, and it is perhaps the most potent of all. . . .

Let's suggest that if a life is equivalent to the time on a 24-hour clock, divided into thirds corresponding to eight-hour segments, then one third of our life is spent sleeping. By the time we turn 30 years of age, we have been sleeping for ten years. And if you extend this out to the number of years you might hope to live – let's say 90 – then by the time you hit that magical age, you will have slept about three decades away! I found that quite an arresting thought, not to mention a bit of a wakeup call. Just imagine at age 90, someone giving you back ten years of the life you've slept away. What a precious gift that would be. And yet we quite willingly fritter our time away.

Just think about the way we live our lives. . . . For the first eight years of life we are essentially non-autonomous children, making very few meaningful choices for ourselves. For the next eight years we will be at a school, probably a school of our parents' choice. And again, we are actually making very few decisions for ourselves. Then finally, by the age of about 16, we are finally making our own choices.

We get to decide whether we carry on at school and then university, or whether we strike out into the world of work. We get to decide whether we shack up with someone, whether we want to travel or settle down. . . .

Looking at it that way, we can see that we have really only been truly living for a very short time by the time we turn 30. Factor in all the other responsibilities that accrue over those 30 years – and all the tedious things like shopping – and you can see how little of our lives we are truly acting on our own free will, living the kind of life we want, freed from societal norms or other people's expectations. I do think that realisation, coupled with all of the other time I'd effectively lost, was the reason I was so desperate to keep finding new things to do with my life.

Having a life-changing accident does obviously help focus the mind. (But if you're reading this and you haven't experienced a life-changing injury, I really don't recommend that you go out and collide with a vehicle like I did; there are much easier ways to find new meaning and purpose in your life!) In my disturbed brain, there was an all-too-linear path proceeding from work, on to retirement, and then on to death. My sense of my own mortality was, unsurprisingly, running rampant. So the imperative to rise again and do meaningful (or at least interesting) things with my life had suddenly shifted into pin-sharp focus. And when I thought about it, there were still too many things that I wanted to be able to do. Goddammit, I was not done yet. I still felt as if I had the capacity to give so much, professionally and personally. There would be plenty of time to sleep when I was done.

More prosaically, I had an exceedingly strong sense of responsibility. I was so grateful for all of the people who had helped me along the way, and I would have felt as if I was diminishing all of their contributions if I did not try to make something more of myself. I also subscribed to the Aristotelean model that if one has an opportunity to flourish and can flourish, then one has a responsibility to do just that. And by Aristotle's definition, to flourish is the highest aim and achievement of human endeavour.

I didn't feel as if I was off to a very promising start. I had arrived in a strange kind of 'nothing time' or what I now had to call my retirement, bearing in mind, of course, that I had not chosen to retire. Nor would I have made that choice given the opportunity. I felt that I was much too young to retire, particularly with having so much still to achieve. If I (or you) asked colleagues or ex-colleagues whether they would like to retire early – specifying that they don't have to endure a crippling accident first – I wonder what they would say. On the one hand, there is the great allure of uncapped leisure time, but again, I wonder how much of a draw that is when all of one's friends and colleague are still working. It's nice to have the time to go and see new places or play sports, but only if there is someone to do those things with who isn't 65+!

Even more significantly, I do believe that work goes on teaching us about humanity: there is a shared responsibility in difficult situations, the camaraderie of sharing difficult times that can be a bonding experience in the workplace, whatever that workplace is. And to be successful at work, we need to work in a team. Every team has its strengths and weaknesses, and to achieve success, we need to accommodate the weakest link in any team. We have to be able to work cooperatively, and that teaches us so much about human interaction. It is work that produces the majority of our friends and, very often, gives us our sense of purpose, helping to satisfy the inherent need to contribute. Going to work provides us with so much more than a just a salary. It helps us to understand what it means to be human. And, of course, we are people of contrasts, and very often we crave work purely because it makes our leisure time that much more meaningful, special, and enjoyable.

Having more time on my hands outside of work, even after I had factored in all of the things I needed to do to maintain my ongoing improvement, didn't help me take any better control over it. Time continued to frustrate and confuse me, and if anything, it seemed to race on ahead of me. Nighttimes alone are surely one of the greatest threats to anyone's sanity, and when my thoughts had a degree of freedom to roam, the unhealthiest recesses of my mind opened up and played merry hell with me.

How do you deal with that? There is no magic bullet answer, except to say: there is no going back. Well, by Christ, that is stating the bloody obvious, but it did me good to remember it sometimes. As I have mentioned before, recovery (such as it is) can be such a jerky, seemingly uncoordinated process that does not progress in a smooth and seamless fashion. The things that made me sad did not merely go away years and years later, and perhaps I would have worried if they had, as if they were still lurking somewhere in my subconscious, waiting to strike when I least expected it.

There remained – and to this day, there remain – a great many things that I could not think about without them producing an extended bout of self-centred and potentially self-destructive melancholy. But even then, even if I forced myself to reflect on them, I could not cry. One of the many things that hurt me to reflect on was the near-meteoric advancement in the world of intensive care medicine. I had been on quite a learning journey from being a physiotherapy student on an Australian intensive care unit ward round to becoming an intensive care consultant in Britain and then an associate professor in medical ethics and law. But that journey had come to an abrupt halt. Whenever I met anyone in person or online and they asked, 'What do you – or did you – do?' I had to embarrassedly tell them that I was retired. And again, I couldn't cry for what I had lost.

I could perhaps have resorted to the final recourse for so many people who are permanently out of work but still have delusions of grandeur. . . . I could have said, 'I am a blogger and author!' (I am thinking of a number of friends here who shall remain nameless.)

You may well have noticed that I started every sentence in that last paragraph with 'I. . .' and yes, I am painfully, acutely aware that my thinking sometimes degenerates into me, me, me. . . . And even that makes me want to cry, and I still can't.

At the top of this list of things that I could not think about was of course – forever and always – my family. If there had been a moment when the source of my anger and frustration and my pain and sadness had moved from the collision to the loss of everything it brought about, I couldn't pinpoint it. But it was always the things that had been forcibly taken from me that hurt the most. Even at the height of my self-absorption, I extrapolated some of the pain I imagined they felt, as well as basking in my own. They had not asked for any of it either, and just like me, they had had to make their own sacrifices too.

They had woken up that morning expecting their lives to carry on as normal. But for them, there was no more normal life after that day. For better or worse there were no more sights of Dad dancing around the table and singing so desperately out of tune, while they all wailed at me to stop as I finished with a big crescendo and hugged their mother. (Just another normal day in the life of a family with a permanently and catastrophically tone-deaf dad!) And those memories – still so very clear to me – are almost unbearably painful. Still I could not cry, and still the clock kept ticking.

But that very ticking of the clock was, in the end, a great motivator, particularly when it came to the dating scene. That was a 'scene' that I had hoped to never have to embrace ever again, nor had I had any expectations of doing so as a happily married family man. But all those very human imperatives remained, and I sought – and was starting to feel as if I deserved – companionship.

If you have ever wanted to find out just how resilient you are, surviving a near-death collision might just classify as slightly easier than subjecting yourself to the dating scene! I could not quite believe how long it took to find a meaningful person, and it just made me feel so ugly and stupid. I knew that everyone's lives that had once been so closely intertwined with mine were moving inexorably ahead with such ease, while mine was resolutely stuck. And after every failed date, I returned to an emptier life than before and sat in front of my computer again, just killing time until I found something – anything – better to do.

I do think that my perspectives on dating had been coloured by my experiences in recovery. As someone who had fought so hard just to achieve any level of physical competence, I couldn't help but be amazed at how little respect some people had for themselves, and I wondered how I could hope or expect to find a life partner who did respect themselves and their own body.

Reader, I will spare you all of the sordid details, but suffice to say, I persevered with dating. And while I doubt there will be too many young ladies crying as they read this, I did find a wonderful woman to share my life with. If anything should reassure you that anything is possible after undergoing the kind of trauma that I did – and perhaps you did – then I hope that does.

I managed to 'trap' a girl despite all of my failings; she still drives me on and actually believes in me. Before any of you rush to call the police to say that I have trapped a beautiful young lady – and you will hear me refer to her as my 'Trappee' – I can assure you that I am only using that term because for so long I could easily have believed that would have been the only way I could ever have found someone again. So don't worry, she has been corralled of her own accord and at her own free will. I do sometimes think those people with their pinkish-purple uniforms and their exceptionably tight-fitting jackets will be coming soon to rescue her from her madness!

It did not matter how well and truly infatuated my Trappee was, I could not help but think how short-changed she must feel by our relationship. How she must notice every little difficulty with everything that I used to be able to do so easily, if not without thinking. While it was true that I could do most of the things I needed to be able to do to live a verging-on-normal life, I needed to concentrate so incredibly hard on them. It's hard to make a spontaneous gesture when tying up your own shoelaces takes so much effort. For me, just turning around to say goodbye to someone felt what I imagined it must be like for a high-wire walker!

When she read this bit, my dear Trappee said, with no little irony, 'So, am I to understand that you feel useless because you cannot turn around to wave goodbye to someone?' I am sure there will be someone in your life that will help to keep you grounded too. Listen to them, even when you don't feel like listening to them. Because they will hold your hand while you totter, step by uncertain step, across the chasm stretching out below the high wire.

It's like I said before, relationships are built upon teamwork. And it was that part of my life that I knew I had been missing for so very long. But with my beloved Trappee, I – or rather we – had invested in the shared responsibility of a relationship. I relished that renewed sense of life being about more than just me. It was a big part of what I had been looking for. Our relationship has brought a sense of shared purpose; just like the functioning of one's brain and body, it relies on a special kind of synergy.

Indeed, the functioning of our body is, as I had learned over ten+ years of struggle, a form of teamwork like no other. For instance, when we cut ourselves, our blood clotting system needs to be working, and our digestive system needs to be working to ensure all of the nutrients are in the right place at the right time. Obviously, our circulatory system needs to be spot on too, so that the clotting factors can get to the area quickly.

My own brain – even what was left of it – had been in desperate need of someone to bounce ideas off, someone to be encouraging. Someone who could shrug off the many, many times I wander off into a period of self-indulgent melancholy. Someone who would still be there waiting for me and still supporting me when I come back from the brink! I sometimes think these are some of the most important behaviours we can model for our children, so that they can grow up in that kind of environment, and then they in turn will do the same things for their children and so on, and so on. That's a kind of immortality worth striving for.

11 How I Learned to Keep Striving for Every Physical and Cognitive Improvement

A Lifetime Later

I have often wondered, what scars I will bear after going through all of this? Perhaps it is a bit like the birth of my first child. As my wife went through the agony of childbirth, I couldn't help but think like a doctor and wonder what the outcome would be for my child and my wife, already worrying about the worst hypoxic brain damage and the complications of preeclampsia. . . . And then, when the screaming had risen to its ear-splitting crescendo, she rolled over and said, 'Well, that wasn't too bad! Shall we have another one?' As if that wasn't enough, the madwife – sorry, midwife – then asked me if I wanted to go around to the business end and cut the cord! No, I did not want to do that, thank you very much. I felt as if we'd both gained enough psychological scars, and I didn't want to add on any visual ones as well.

I suppose that tells us that it's almost impossible to get through life without a few scars, and maybe that's not such a bad thing. The psychological scars of childbirth must be worth it, after all; my wife went through it twice more. I never did cut any cords though! So maybe, like her, I've started to learn to wear my scars with pride.

And as I reflect on that, I am very reluctant to say this is the final chapter because it isn't *my* final chapter! What feels like a lifetime later, I am just as reluctant to face up to the fact that my body is still so bloody buggered. It has gone from being able to win the odd tennis match to being

DOI: 10.4324/9781003244370-12

a bloody dodgy body that, while it can do most things, it mostly bloody won't. It's galling to think that I will still have to be doing my random exercises well into my sixties, and gee, can you guess, I am pretty desperate to use some more strident language here. My fifties are going the same way as my forties. My scars haven't faded yet.

So it won't surprise you to know that I could have called this chapter, 'How I Learned to Survive the Wrist-Slitting Years' to describe the time that has passed since that day. It honestly feels like a lifetime since I was standing on the start line in my gimp suit, with a whole heap of other rubber gimps lined up for the triathlon. There I was, an NHS consultant in intensive care medicine, the associate professor of medical law and ethics, a happily married man and father to three children, and all it took was five seconds to obliterate all of it. I effectively died on the operating table, and if it hadn't been for my friend and colleague with the defibrillator, I would have died when I went into cardiac arrest.

I know that five years, ten years, or 14.9 years are all equally arbitrary markers of time, but as I think I've indicated, the passage of time matters, particularly when you feel the pressure of making the most of whatever time is left. More than that, it helps us check in on our progress in a more objective way. Even when it seemed as if my progress moved at a glacial pace, I could see what I had accomplished over a span of months and years, and that was, in some small way, helpful.

In the time since the collision, I had witnessed the loss of myself as an independent and private adult. I had effectively lost my family, and I had absolutely lost my wife. And at first, I was seemingly helpless to do anything about any of it. I was, to all intents and purposes, locked in stasis, like a dispassionate or disinterested observer watching an unstoppable force tear through my life and then raking over the embers of whatever was left.

My catalogue of tragedies was all witnessed by a succession of well-meaning strangers. And as difficult as that was for me at times, I was – and remain – incredibly grateful to every one of them. Indeed, if I think about them now, I still well up at the memories of those people and those times.

There are dangers with looking back too often. How easy it is to get stuck in the past, lost in the sheer bloody misery of it all. At the height of my wrist-slitting years, there was a seductive pull to ruminating endlessly over it all. And I spent my fair share of hours in the past, bitterly regretting the events of that day and pining for what was and could never be again. But looking back also encourages us to look forward and helps us recontextualise where we're going. It was only really when I felt as if I was in some way back to myself and felt able to carve out a new life, with new meaning, that I was really able to think beyond myself. I still wanted to find ways to help others or at least provide something that might have meaning or significance to people.

That's the thing about life, I suppose; existing is all very well, but you know when you're in some way recovered because merely existing is not enough anymore. I have always believed in a meritocracy, and I was bloody determined to get back to some sort of emeritus life or at least a life worthy of merit. It was as much for my kids as it was for me. Like that thought I had when I left for the triathlon, I wanted to lead by example. Back then, I wanted them to see how the hard work of training had paid off. That didn't actually go so well, as you know! But I knew that I could now lead by example in an unambiguously positive way.

I was invited to give a lecture to a stroke group, and I knew that so much of what I had experienced in terms of reimagining life after a debilitating intervention would help. Here is some of what I prepared for them:

While it will become much more difficult to learn new skills, I am definitely not saying that you cannot ever learn a new skill. True, you can expect to find it incredibly hard to develop new abilities you did not have before your accident or your stroke, such as standing to put on your shoes and socks. And even when it comes to doing things you have always done, such as buttering your toast with your affected hand, you may find that these finer skills will also take a little longer to master. However, the brain is a pretty amazing thing when you think about it – which is in itself something I haven't been able to do until recently. After my accident, it took some time before I was really able to think with any conviction, and when you regain an ability like that, you truly appreciate how amazing it is.

There are approximately 67 billion neurons up there, well, there are in yours anyway, maybe not in mine anymore! And there are countless more connections as well, and if you follow this to its logical conclusion then it is absolutely amazing to think that we came from nothing. Our brains have developed from nothing at all, just happenstance and the circumstantial meeting of atoms, and then these atoms just happened to twitch into life.

Putting it all into perspective, 'all' it takes to be able to learn a new skill or to re-learn an old one is to put down some new connections. What is different about my brain? Well, I have become acutely or suddenly stupid, thick as mince, you might say! Also, I have countless neurons switched on and opposing the neurons which are correctly attempting to complete a given task. In other words, these auxiliary neurons are working against me, i.e., they are unhelpfully activating muscles that oppose the muscles that are correctly attempting to complete a task. My body has become like my wife . . . it can do it, but it just bloody won't!

And by the way, no, I have not always had a servant dedicated to buttering my toast. And no, I was not born with a silver spoon in my mouth either. In fact,

I remember my mother telling us, over and over again, how we had always had what we needed, even if we had not always had what we wanted, which obviously begs the question: based on whose assessment?! It may well be that I have become a little bit more obstreperous now. I'm sure my mother had it easy with me as her son, but with time comes cynicism and a tiny bit of obstreperousness. Even cantankerousness! But not any loss of determination, and it is determination that will serve you so well when you are on your rehab plan. Just think of all of those neurons up there, and all the connections that are just waiting to form a new pathway to achieving a new goal. . . .

Perhaps I should have told them how every second I was up there, I was paranoid about falling over, and if they'd been underwhelmed by my less-than-dramatic delivery, then it might have been because I was concentrating so damned hard on just standing up, rather than what I was saying. I could have told them how hard it was for me to walk and talk on the phone at the same time. I can't even walk and chew gum, so thank goodness my parents instilled a dislike for chewing gum.

But I do think I was able to prove by example that in spite of what one may think when the task seems so gargantuan, there is a way back from most situations. Perhaps that reflects how much of an optimist I am in that I was even then – perhaps even now – still waiting for my attributes to miraculously come back. So if it sounds like I had it all figured out and was absolutely positively out of the woods, you'd be only half right.

I'm not sure if I'll ever be entirely out of the woods. More likely I'll carry on skirting the edge of the woods with occasional forays deeper under the canopy and then out into the clearing. And if I was giving that speech now, I might also have wanted to tell my audience, as they hung attentively on every word I said, how recovery – whatever that is – isn't really an end point. There will never be a moment when I'm signed off as 'recovered,' just as there'll never be a time when I don't have regrets or anguish or when I don't feel like railing against the sheer bloody injustice of it all.

In a bleaker moment after I gave that speech – when to all intents and purposes, I was 'better' – I blogged about how my life had been for diddly-squat. A friend responded, saying how they'd studied at Cambridge and Harvard; done a range of amazing roles and had amazing responsibilities; managed $100+ million in other people's money; knew many millionaires and billionaires . . . but still didn't have a job! They said they hadn't experienced anything like I'd experienced, and yet selfishly said the same thing: 'What has my life amounted to? It's all for naught.'

They knew, objectively, that their thinking was flawed; they could rattle off their expertise in disciplines from engineering to law to finance. They could see the absolute metrics of their own success, and yet it didn't seem to matter. They went on:

'Think of the hundreds of people's lives you directly impacted as a doctor and (most fundamentally) as a mutual member of our common man: all your countless patients, your fellow doctors, your students, family and friends across the globe – astounding! You've made a profound impact on the world! I use your example of outright determination, hard work and conviction to achieve; I use that example, your (!) example with my kids and others all the time, to inspire greatness in others . . . and it works!

'I openly admit that I am fundamentally incapable of understanding/comprehending what you've been through. But (in my humble opinion) it is that unfathomably unique experience that you can contribute to the world and much more . . . whether through documenting your life, educational/

teaching work, a book about your experience, or something different again.'

So what did I say in return? Well, obviously I was exceedingly grateful, and I did wonder if their words were really meant for me or for some other angelic demigod! But I did say I would endeavour to live up to their words – and meant it.

I wondered how one could be an inspiration doing nothing at all. I suppose Gandhi would have something to say about that! But I really did feel as if anything I was doing was less for a great cause than out of simple necessity. And it didn't matter if my friends told me that I was inspirational, because I still wanted more. Can you believe it?

Earlier, I talked about the perspective that passing time can afford us. It did worry me so much that I was letting time slip through my fingers, but I do believe that documenting my own progress helped me. Perhaps it could help you too? So often, it may appear as if we are standing still as the world moves on without us. Or swaying ever so slightly side to side as I used to do in the early days of recovery. It is only when we read back over our own journey that we appreciate that we have been moving right along with everyone else, albeit in our own unique way.

There are still things that surprise me about the journey I've been on. Take my arm. No, please take it! Despite it being many years since I had full, unrestricted movement in my left arm, I'm still constantly amazed or, at the very least, constantly pleased that I have two arms, and every time I get to use my left arm, I sort of smile to myself that I can do it. At the beginning, I really did write it off as ever being any use to me at all. I remember consigning myself to a life of only ever using my right hand and giving up on my left completely, not to mention giving up on shaving! I hated only ever being able to give the wettest and weakest of handshakes. But not anymore! I've come a long way from having to ask people to cut up my food in a restaurant so that I could eat with my kids. And now I'm always looking for more things that I can do using my left arm and hand. I even started drumming to develop more independence and coordination between my arms. And I'm pleased to say that I am able to eat about as politely as any Australian ever could.

When I look back, there are more of those positive reflections than I ever would have thought possible. I still sometimes stop and reflect with quiet joy on not having to be in a wheelchair anymore. I do still have seemingly insurmountable challenges; I still rue the time lost with my children and the difference between the father I was and the father I am. Though I suppose you'd have to ask the children how they reflect on that! And it's strange to think that in their minds, I have mostly always been like this!

The quest for suitably fulfilling work goes on. Maybe I will make it as a life coach. Or a writer. Maybe there is another path waiting to be explored.

The important thing is to keep buggering on, eh? Grudgingly, I can say that the fortitude that has brought me – and you, I suspect – this far has outweighed so many of the losses I have incurred. I didn't give up on my arm, or my reading, or my memory, or my tennis, or any of it. For the most part, I did not outwardly show the pain I was enduring – and that's not to say that I couldn't have done – and I carried on being me. Perhaps it shows the extent of my fortitude; perhaps it just proves once and for all that I was always a miserable old git, and no one even noticed the change!

I found a way of surviving that was uniquely mine. Andrew Tillyard AD may not be the finest specimen to walk this green earth, but by God, he is a survivor. And so are you. I do think uniqueness – mine and yours – is a hugely valuable commodity here. We each need to find a way of achieving the recovery that works for us. I came up with an analogy about brain injury that sums it all up to me in a way that – having been through it – makes sense. In this analogy, we can think of our brain as an apartment or flat. The old way of thinking was that a brain injury is a bit like losing the keys to your flat. The keys represent a function of the brain that lets you in. Simple enough. The flat still exists, but without the keys, you can't access it in the way you used to be able to.

Early on in recovery, you come up against dead ends or road work that makes it even more difficult for you to access your flat, and it used to be thought that after a brain injury we would never get our keys back. They were lost. Gone. We were essentially told that we had to get over that fact and move on. But I didn't want a life of shinnying up a drainpipe and forcing my way through a half-open window! And from my own experience, I don't think it's like that. I believe that the keys are still out there somewhere, and instead of going on trying to find alternatives, we should redouble our efforts at finding the keys that unlock everything. It takes an awful lot of time and hard work, of course, I can vouch for that. In my own recovery, I have gone from a brain-dead kumquat who made a goldfish look like a Mensa candidate to being able to remember eight random words, and I can do almost everything the experts said I would never be able to do, including reading and typing, let alone writing a book!

Talking of which, I was quite worried about finding the right way to end this book. After all, this is not the end for me. There is still so much for me to achieve, and as I have said there is no going backwards in this life. So, let's call this an interim report. My own assessment suggests that I continue to feel guilty because I used to have a career and a truly independent life. Sure, I am completely independent now in terms of being able to look after myself, but I still have so much further to go until I am remotely near to anything I could do before as Andrew BC. There's no getting around the fact that I am less than him. I do not have the same physical abilities as he did. I still do not have a career or even a job which would enable me to be generous towards my Trappee and my family, who have all been so incredibly generous towards or at least tolerant of me and all my requirements, which are legion now.

I have missed being able to think of myself as someone who was capable of inducing pride in others and in myself. I will go on trying to prove to myself that Andrew AD is capable and worthy of respect. It is, inevitably, so much worse trying to prove anything to myself; I can tell you that I am a very, very hard taskmaster! There have been times when I have missed Andrew BC very much. I know that I could go on trying to match him – and failing for the rest of my life – but that would only put me under an undue and unnecessary pressure. At some point I had to draw a line in the sand and say: I am not the man I was. And I have to focus on what I can do. . . .

I still have people to strive for, other than me. So I do things in the knowledge that they matter to my children, to my Trappee, my friends, and the people that I still feel I can offer tangible help to. In the frustration that comes of knowing that I cannot simply step back into a career or a life where I could quite simply achieve so much of what I want, there is the impetus to go on striving.

In short – and forgive me for getting a bit evangelical here – I will not rest until I have achieved the three pillars that I believe make a life that is worthwhile. First and foremost, there is a family, then there is having a significant other, such as my Trappee, and lastly there is having a career.

For now, this book will have to do! And perhaps it will allow me to feel just a little bit of that pride that I have been missing in my life. I am one who has defied the experts. And it's worth reiterating here that experts, as well as any of us, just have to guess sometimes. Don't ever let the word of an expert put you off striving for more. So many of the experts that you and I will have dealt with are working in a field that is still relatively poorly understood. And so I say again – with a slightly glib tongue – that some of them might as well be considered experts in magic or in levitating. I would suggest that you keep that to yourself, but actually, you could say as much to many, many experts in medicine and they will wholeheartedly agree with you. What they do know is broad and impressive, but it still only scratches the grey, undulating surface of the human brain!

Recovery, as I have come to understand it, is a baffling and unpredictable thing. People can achieve so much more than would have ever been thought possible. And perhaps now, my own experience will give people a little more knowledge about brain injury and, even more importantly, some greater hope.

The key to it, as far as I can see, is just perseverance and determination. It is never, ever accepting that you have lost the keys to your flat. It is trying new things; it is doing whatever it takes to make one simple improvement, in the knowledge that one improvement can so often lead to so many others.

Afterword – A Happy Ending?

If my story has seemed at times to focus on the negative, it is only because I sometimes think that the greatest trauma of all was not the accident itself, but rather the response to it.

Let me explain what I mean. First, there was the injury itself. So far, so traumatic, you might think. But the second hit of trauma was altogether more insidious. It was all to do with the complete lack of understanding around the possibility of recovery from the injury. Indeed, my family and my colleagues were told that I was essentially done for. At first, they were told that I would never recover. Then that was revised to suggest that any recovery I did make would be mostly confined to the first one or two years post-trauma.

Well, sure, at the time of writing, it has taken me nearly ten years to get to a point where I feel as if I am getting closer – in many ways – to where I was before the trauma. But I have continued to improve. And I *continue* to improve.

So there is a happy ending. Of that I am in no doubt. Even though I did, in every meaningful way, lose everything that I had, I have since found new direction in life, and I have found myself. *Am I Still Me?* Yes, I think I am. Even a non-nonsense Australian would admit that's worth a tear of joy. But, like so many of the best endings, it is tinged with a hint of melancholy. . . .

Just imagine what my life might have looked like if someone – anyone – had simply said: 'More extensive recovery is possible, but it is going to take some time. Don't give up on him.' If they had, I think that there might have been quite a different outcome for me and for my family.

I wonder if every one of us who faces a life-altering incident on this scale has to navigate a kind of double trauma. And I wonder how much more we could all achieve if only we were given more hope that recovery is possible.

So, to all of you out there reading this, I will simply say, never give up. Have hope. Whatever else deserts you, cling onto hope like a life raft. Because hope has carried me further than conventional wisdom would ever have believed possible. It can carry you too.

Pandemic poetry
Will I live will I die?

Will I live will I die I breathe in and out

But it is not me the incessant bleep bleep of the saturation monitor mirrored by the nurse's eyes thank god for her eyes

Thank god for her eyes will I make it will I die and everyone is looking at me: will I make it will I be and still I cannot touch my family. a tear rolls down my face but no one notices the pain I feel inside and I think I can see the abject exhaustion on my family's faces: silently I Say goodbye my friend goodbye my lover

My god what have I done to them what have I put them through another day.

Another evening is survived; will I live will I die;

My chest raises up but it is not me, as the ventilator breathes in for me. another day survived another evening to come I am not done and on it goes

Climate poetry – trees I look you're not there I look and you're not there

I breathe I breathe you shade me you remove the city scape green the city my first love scribbled into your trunk. what have I done why have I been so lazy? Oh my god what have I done for you. the lost land the lost houses the lost islands. You are not there you are not there. it is not a matter of a museum not being there it is AN entire species it is our planet

for what a cheap flight or a cheap holiday. the lost species: insects dolphins

Trees I breathe I breathe you shade me, my first kiss.

my first snog, pencil writing desk I breathe

cemetery, I become you

Geography Roots erosion, paper, desks chairs history: the endeavour cutty sark Vikings the new world medicine

Houses become homes: history physiology medicine geography. Nutrition

Trees: I breathe I breathe you shade me.

my first kiss my first snog my first love

pencil writing desk I breathe

Roots erosion, pencils and paper. chairs history medicine geography physiology I breathe

history the endeavour cutty sark Vikings the new world houses become homes history physiology; I breathe medicine geography. Nutrition, fruit and vegetables,

my first kiss my first snog my first love

pencil writing desk I breathe

Roots erosion, pencils and paper. chairs history medicine geography physiology I breathe

history the endeavour cutty sark Vikings the new world
houses become homes history physiology; I breathe
medicine geography. Nutrition, fruit and vegetables,

Climate poetry

Is this my legacy for you I am so sorry what have I done
to you or for you oh my god what was once green and
pleasant is now barren and arid

it is

I am so sorry

is this my legacy for you is this my legacy for you I am
so sorry?

why did I ignore all of the signals, what have I done to
you. or what have I done for you why when the earth
was burning why did I not do anything. Oh my god
I look up and see the desert when I could do something
I did not do anything or everything I could. But now
I have left you nothing no leeway. no slack at all for
your mum and dad and that is not saying anything about
the animals

Index

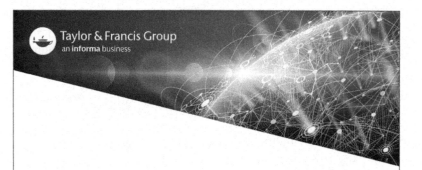